MW00358411

A WELL MIND

Lisa Parkinson Roberts has worked in the field of health and nutrition for over a decade, and has a PhD in Nutrition Science. Her work has been published extensively and she has presented her research at both local and international nutrition conferences.

Lisa aims to bring the public a comprehensive, accessible overview of nutrition advice. Having suffered mental illness for most of her life, she now enjoys a different state of mind and is passionate about helping others to do the same.

Visit **www.lisaparkinsonroberts.com** to find out more.

A WELL MIND

~

The tools for attaining mental wellbeing

LISA PARKINSON ROBERTS, PH.D.

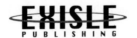

First published 2021

Exisle Publishing Pty Ltd
PO Box 864, Chatswood, NSW 2057, Australia
226 High Street, Dunedin, 9016, New Zealand
www.exislepublishing.com

Copyright © 2021 in text: Lisa Parkinson Roberts

Lisa Parkinson Roberts asserts the moral right to be identified as the author of this work.

All rights reserved. Except for short extracts for the purpose of review, no part of this book may be reproduced, stored in a retrieval system or transmitted in any form or by any means, whether electronic, mechanical, photocopying, recording or otherwise, without prior written permission from the publisher.

A CiP record for this book is available from the National Library of Australia.

ISBN 978-1-925820-78-2

Designed by Enni Tuomisalo

Typeset in Palatino, 10.5pt.

Printed in China

This book uses paper sourced under ISO 14001 guidelines from well-managed forests and other controlled sources.

10 9 8 7 6 5 4 3 2 1

Disclaimer
This book is a general guide only and should never be a substitute for the skill, knowledge and experience of a qualified medical professional dealing with the facts, circumstances and symptoms of a particular case. The nutritional, medical and health information presented in this book is based on the research, training and professional experience of the author, and is true and complete to the best of their knowledge. However, this book is intended only as an informative guide; it is not intended to replace or countermand the advice given by the reader's personal physician. Because each person and situation is unique, the author and the publisher urge the reader to check with a qualified healthcare professional before using any procedure where there is a question as to its appropriateness. The author, publisher and their distributors are not responsible for any adverse effects or consequences resulting from the use of the information in this book. It is the responsibility of the reader to consult a physician or other qualified healthcare professional regarding their personal care. The intent of the information provided is to be helpful; however, there is no guarantee of results associated with the information provided.

For Indigo and Ziggy
(and other grandchildren to come).

May your heart be full and your mind well.

CONTENTS

Preface

For most of my life, a well mind was a foreign concept to me. From my earliest memories I felt I had no control over my mental health and simply had to play the cards I was dealt.

As an adult I became interested in the idea of mental wellness, as opposed to mental illness, as a result of my personal struggle to attain a well mind (and it has been a long, hard-fought struggle).

I was first diagnosed with bipolar disorder at the age of fifteen. I had visited a doctor because I thought I was pregnant. During the consultation he picked up on symptoms (apparently I wasn't making any sense and babbling about things he didn't understand). I believed the doctor was telling me I was crazy: and I was sure he was the crazy one. I was living away from home at the time and so couldn't be prescribed medication without my parents' consent. I didn't want to tell anyone, and I certainly did not want to believe I had a mental illness.

Here is a little more context. At the time I was occasionally visiting an evangelical church. I suppose I was searching for God because I felt so lost. One Sunday night there was a sermon during which psychiatric illness was discussed. There I was sitting wide eyed on the edge of my seat as I was informed that mental illness (like the one I apparently had) was a symptom of a demon living inside of me. Can you imagine? I already felt like I was bad news, without everyone believing I had demons inside of me as well. And so, I ignored the doctor the first time, and stuck my head deeply in the sand.

That was the first of several diagnoses I have received, ranging from bipolar disorder, to depression, to OCD.

Although there were times I was so unwell in my mind it's miraculous I am still here to tell the story, there were other times I have just had a tough time getting out of bed, felt anxious, or just a general malaise.

I have learned an important lesson during my journey: struggle can alchemize into growth, and we all struggle; the struggle just presents differently for each of us.

I now manage my mind and keep it well by using food as medicine and adopting a variety of tools — tools I want to share with you. I know this is possible because I am doing it.

A question I have often pondered is why we are taught how to care only for our body and not our mind. This is slowly changing, but more in the context of 'Better do crosswords and talk to people daily so we don't get Alzheimer's,' or 'Better see a doctor if I'm feeling depressed.'

Imagine if in school we had lessons on cultivating a well mind. Imagine being given tools to calm our nervous system, tools to ward off anxiety and depression, foods to nourish and heal our mind. Imagine if we were taught that we are *not* our thoughts; rather, we are an audience who has the power to choose which thoughts to watch and nurture, and which thoughts to dismiss. Imagine if we were taught how to rewrite the narrative in our head, and let go of what doesn't serve us. If we were taught to just be still. Our world would be much calmer.

We don't have to imagine — it can be a reality. There is much research in this area highlighting that food and positive lifestyle choices promote mental wellness: they are grounded in science and they are easy to access.

When working on my PhD in nutrition and sensory science, I explored the effects of a compound in food on inflammation in human muscle cells. During this time I saw first-hand the positive effects that a phenolic compound (found in virgin olive oil), exerted on inflammatory processes. This led to the realisation of an intimate relationship between three elements: nutrients found in our food, inflammation, and the health of our body and brain. I have since been on a journey to reduce inflammation in my body and mind, and have incorporated several mind-changing strategies into my own life.

An important point to share with you is that before I could get to a place of being able to invest the effort required to change my mind (It's health — not shifting decisions from smashed-avocado toast to a chicken salad!), I had to *believe* that the effort would pay off. And I had to reflect on why the health of my mind was so important. This is similar to a person embarking on a weight-loss journey, or a lifestyle overhaul to create a healthy body. It takes time, reflection and effort, as well as a large degree of experimentation. I had to get to the point where I believed that a healthy and well mind was a possibility. The small ember of hope that my mind could be considered well caught fire as I observed the changes in myself over time. That fire is growing, and I want others — you — to feel the same.

One of my aims in this book is to drive home the idea that we don't have to be ashamed about feeling hopeless, overwhelmed, sad, unmotivated, irritable, angry, depressed, flat, lethargic, anxious, panicked or crazy (or any other adjective you care to apply). Of course we are likely to feel those things sometimes, but it doesn't have to steal our joy, impact our lives or engulf us with shame.

Another aim is to introduce the importance of a well mind and provide the tools we can use to promote the health and wellbeing of our mind and emotions. The beauty of a well mind is that it alters the landscape surrounding us. We can move from living in the past, and with it anxiety and regret, or from being caught up in the future, and with it uncertainty, to experiencing each day mindfully and calmly.

I always desired to feel well in my mind, but a state of being calm, content and centred seemed so unobtainable for someone like me. I have to pinch myself sometimes when I exert control over my reactions, and feel that my mind has reached a healthy and well state that I hadn't previously dreamed possible. The things I have learned along the way to a well mind will come through on these pages. And the beautiful thing is, it works. It requires effort, but it does work.

And so, I have written this book for you; to help you alleviate malaise in your mind, and to impart the message that you have more control over the wellbeing of your mind than you might currently believe.

As Ernest Agyemang Yeboah suggests:

From dawn to the time you retire, your mind can be a very good friend to you and your mind can also be your worst friend. What goes into your mind each day becomes your friend so mind your mind![1]

Throughout these pages I share my own personal stories, and stories from others so that we can journey together on the path to a well mind and be the best version of us we can be.

Introduction

'We are what our thoughts have made us; so take care about what you think. Words are secondary. Thoughts live; they travel far.'

Swami Vivekananda[2]

It *is* possible to achieve wellness in your mind. I should know: I have lived it.

Now, you may not feel that your mind is 'unwell', but if you are reading this book, I suspect that you have had moments when you ponder the possibility of feeling better emotionally and mentally. If so, this book is for you.

First, a bit about me.

From memory, my first encounter with an unwell mind occurred when I was just fourteen years old. I had a vague understanding that my mind wasn't 'normal' because often I couldn't keep track of my thoughts, and would imagine the most dreadful, frightening things. Things I was sure never set foot in the minds of my friends. But at that age I had more important things to worry about. There were raging hormones swirling around my young body, school work to focus on, boys to catch my interest and friends to occupy my time. My sugar intake was high, sleep cycles were becoming irregular, and I started to experience hallucinations, paranoia and intense levels of irritability.

On one occasion I began to hear a distinct voice in my head, and then my mind raced out of control. Thoughts grew faster and louder, similar to when you are in a crowded restaurant and everyone is determined to be heard over the noise and so the volume keeps going up and up. My thoughts were battling for attention, they all wanted to be heard. Every thought felt desperately important in that moment and as they screamed for my attention. I couldn't catch even a few of them — let alone all. I couldn't sleep for days, and then I took a nose dive into dark depression where I stayed for a while, until I started to feel an overwhelming energy and everything sped up again.

After that initiation I became more reckless and impulsive, at times depressed and lost. I was drinking, smoking, lying, and often in trouble. I had an affair with a 30-year-old man and was spending my weekends at a local nightclub where he worked as security. I wasn't sleeping or functioning, and soon I left home and got a job (my parents were devastated).

I put myself in terribly dangerous situations and had no regard for myself or others. I simply cheated and lied my way out of unsavoury situations when I could. I met the man who would become my husband and then my ex-husband (still my friend), when I was just thirteen (he was seventeen), and I fell pregnant and married him when I was just seventeen. Our second child was born when I was eighteen, ten months after our first.

For almost 30 years I cycled between feeling depressed, anxious, manic and irritable (sometimes stable). My mind has been replete with irrational and racing thoughts, chaotic emotions and paranoia (always feeling sure someone is out to get me, lie to me, hurt me — I have even imagined people were trying to kill me).

There have been many times when feelings of grandeur have overwhelmed any logical sense of reason. In those moments I was special and had important things to teach the world. I had grandiose delusions, jealous delusions, paranoid delusions ... all kinds of delusions. Fortunately, I felt I was so special that only someone as special as me would understand. So, I kept notes about my deep connection with God and my understanding of all things mystical; rather than sharing this wonderful news with the world.

At my lowest I would drop my kids to school, go home and cycle out of control, sometimes spending the entire day curled up in the foetal position in my wardrobe. I would throw things, hurt myself, cry and rage all day. Then, I would act as normally as I possibly could at school pick-up, or when visitors arrived. Hallucinations were frequent and fear was a constant companion.

This is difficult to share. One day forever etched in my mind was when my children were young and I was doing some shopping on a busy street. Thankfully, I didn't have my kids with me. Thoughts were hurtling out of control as usual — I couldn't slow them down and had been trying for days. I watched people as they passed me, hallucinating that they were all laughing at me as I walked along. It wasn't a jovial laugh, rather a sneering, evil laugh: it filled me with terror. I saw a bus coming towards me, and the urge to jump out in front of it was all too much. I lunged at it expecting to be hit, but instead I tripped and fell — I think. As I sat on the ground sobbing, a man stopped and asked if I was okay. I looked around and saw that people were staring at me as they passed. I was crying uncontrollably and just sat on the pavement completely broken. I have no idea how long I was there. More people had stopped and I was aware of a hand reaching to help me up: I just yelled at them to leave me alone, and then I hysterically ran away.

This particular incident occurred on the main street of the town that I had grown up in. I knew many people in that town, so during the months following I was completely cloaked in shame and paranoia. I was certain that everyone was talking about me and that they knew what a fruit loop I really was. I didn't talk to my husband or anyone because I was terrified I would be put away in a mental hospital and would lose my kids.

Thoughts of jumping in front of moving vehicles (or other dramatic modes to leave this earth) have visited occasionally over the years. Looking back, I don't believe I was truly serious or I would have succeeded; my children were my world and gave me hope. But it's hard to reflect on that objectively, even now.

> ~
>
> A note on suicidal thoughts. If you are suicidal or have entertained thoughts about ending it all, please talk to someone — a friend, family member, health practitioner or counsellor — immediately. And remember this: ceasing to live doesn't remove your pain (you are dead); it actually transfers your pain to the people who love and care about you. To be human is to feel pain, and the pain doesn't last forever.

Obviously I was mentally unwell. I felt I was out of sync with the rest of the world, but fortunately I gravitated towards healthy food and exercise (vanity possibly had something to do with that). It's possible that those healthful habits may have prevented me from reaching rock bottom too many times. However, if I knew back then what I know now, I am sure I would have managed the health of my mind far more effectively.

I'd like to ask you to consider for a moment if your mind is well. Do you have emotional and mental health? Or do you feel that because you don't have a 'mental illness' like I have had, you have no need to think about your mind?

It's an interesting question to ponder. Think about this: just because you're not suffering from heart disease, you still have to take care of your heart. The same is true for your mind. Do we really need to reach rock bottom before we do the work required to achieve a healthy and well mind? Not always, but mostly yes. Why do so many of us need to be beaten into submission before we realise we need to find a way to feel better? Perhaps it's so we can appreciate the reward of working towards mental wellness, whereas if we didn't struggle internally it wouldn't be such a big deal. Perhaps we need to hit the wall enough times to start looking for a door — one door is the tools I share in this book.

~

William James,[3] a noted early American psychologist and philosopher, frequently climbed into bed depressed. He wrote a book, *The Varieties of Religious Experience*, in which he divided humankind into two categories: those who are 'once born' and those who are 'twice born ... the sick souls'.

Once born

The 'once born' are those who make like Julie Andrews, twirling on the meadow in Salzburg. They are predisposed to happiness. They appear to not judge, grumble, fear or complain. There is not an ounce of negativity in their bones and seemingly they skip through life, not bothered by the intense sufferings in the world. They are positive and uplifting souls *all the time*! Okay, I may be a little envious, but I have yet to meet one.

Born again

Now on the other end of the 'hills are alive' stick are those who feel that the world is not so great. They are the twice born. James describes them as:

'persons whose existence is little more than a series of zigzags, as now one tendency and now another gets the upper hand. Their spirit wars with their flesh, they wish for incompatibles, wayward impulses interrupt their most deliberate plans, and their lives are one long drama of repentance and of effort to repair misdemeanours and mistakes.'[4]

Oh dear! However, James expands on this and writes, *'The process is one of redemption, not of mere reversion to natural health, and the sufferer, when saved, is saved by what seems to him a second birth, a deeper kind of conscious being than he could enjoy before.'*

If you search for William James on the Pursuit of Happiness website[5] you will find a clear summary of what James was referring to: the explanation is that the twice-born 'sick souls' are in fact, the lucky ones. This is because the depressed state leads them to smash on rock bottom, from where they can, with some work, 'rise like a phoenix from the ashes' and reach a 'new and higher plane'. The 'sick souls' find more profound happiness and consciousness than they could have experienced if they had cruised through life happy and satisfied. It takes work, but this new 'higher plane' is worth the work.

PART 1:
BECAUSE WE ARE HUMAN

CHAPTER 1:

Shame

'You are imperfect, you are wired for struggle,
but you are worthy of love and belonging.'

Brené Brown[6]

A feeling I am intimately familiar with is shame. Throughout my youth and early adulthood, I lacked control over my emotions. I have experienced screaming meltdowns many times; on the street, in my neighbourhood, in my home, not caring who witnessed the ugly pandemonium flowing from my mouth. It felt so good to unleash the mayhem within, but then shame would descend and I would angrily justify my behaviour.

It's embarrassing to think back to some of the scenes that make up my story. But I have worked hard to get to a place of knowing that my past doesn't define me, nor does my struggle with mental health and wellbeing — just as your past and struggles don't define you.

When I was working in academia teaching nutrition and physiology I felt I was drowning in shame: I didn't feel adequate to be teaching my students health-related content when my mind was so utterly broken. Often I felt so inferior and tarnished because my mind 'came out of the box' broken, rather than 'normal'.

The shame we feel when we don't behave appropriately or if we don't live up to societal norms can be debilitating. We need to overcome the sense of shame so we can move forward. And to get past shame we must employ self-care.

Self-care is crucial and can be defined as any activity that is deliberately adopted to take care of our mental, emotional and physical health. The health of our mind and our emotions is of fundamental importance because our mind and emotions dictate how we feel, how we behave and how we interact with the world. If we have a healthy and well mind, we are more likely to practise self-care and be able to relate to others in a healthy way.

An important point: you don't feel shame when you have the flu; rather you simply take care of your body until it passes. We need to care for our mind rather than heaping shame onto ourselves when its health is letting us down.

Shame changes the way we see ourselves, and this in turn can have a profound impact on our relationships. The saying is true, others can't love us until we love ourselves with all our imperfections.

Shame drives us to view ourselves in a negative light, and the antidote to shame is to accept ourselves warts and all. Difficult to do: we are so tough on ourselves.

A note: the sense of shame can be a result of mental illness and can also contribute to mental illness, in particular depression and anxiety.[7]

So, leave shame behind now, whatever your circumstances, and accept that you are worthy of self-care. Whether you are currently suffering in your mind, or just want to feel the best you can, my words here are to guide you to care for your mind. To protect and heal your mind is the goal.

Before we move on, I want to stress that I am not downplaying the severity of mental-health disorders — not at all. I have been in the depths of mental hell and have clawed my way back. I don't take mental illness lightly, but I believe we possess a degree of control over how we feel in our mind — and I want to help you take control.

What is mental wellness?

Of course, possessing a well mind also connotes the lack of degenerative diseases of the brain, such as Alzheimer's, or other dementias. However, those diseases are not at the heart of this exploration, so I don't discuss neurological pathologies in this book.

Now, you might think that the prevalence of diagnosed mental illness is rapidly shooting up; I did. Actually, it's not. According to data from the Institute of Health Metrics and Evaluation (IHME) derived from the Global Burden of Disease study, there has been little change in the incidence of mental illness since 1990. Perhaps we feel that the prevalence is increasing because we are talking about mental health now, which is great — but talking does not solve the issue. Regardless of the static state, the extent of poor mental health is huge, with 970 million people suffering from a mental or substance-use disorder in 2017.[8] Those kinds of statistics are alarming and indicative of much suffering and mental pain. But how has it reached that level of significance?

We will explore this question throughout the book.

We must also consider that although serotonin is an important neurotransmitter and plays a role in how we feel in our mind, there is no clear way to measure serotonin in the brain; we don't know if blood measures of serotonin reflect brain levels of serotonin. In regards to depression, if a chemical imbalance is responsible for depression, then why don't the treatments that target the neurotransmitters (Selective Serotonin Reuptake Inhibitors or SSRI) work for everyone? And why don't they work faster? The health and wellness of our mind is a complex interaction of several factors.

We are generally exposed to mental illness in the media and public health campaigns, but what about mental *wellness*? What does it mean to be mentally well in the 21st century? Is mental wellness simply the same as not having a mental illness? Physical wellness can be described as taking care of our bodies for optimal health and functioning. I propose that the definition of mental wellness is taking care of our minds to achieve the same: optimal health and functioning. Before we meander through some tools needed for mental wellness, let's discuss the stigma associated with mental suffering.

Stigma and power

After the birth of her first child, Beth suffered terrible mental anguish. She would be woken by her crying newborn and then drown in a sense of dread. She didn't think she could get through another day. Beth had experienced anxiety in previous years but had never considered that she might be susceptible to post-natal depression.

Beth had what others would consider the perfect life. She had had a successful career, met and fell in love with a wonderful man, fell pregnant easily, and didn't have the financial pressure of getting straight back to work after her maternity leave ended.

The first two weeks were fine; she and baby bonded beautifully. But after her husband went back to work, things started to slide downhill fast. She was soon obsessing over whether everything was sterile enough for her newborn, whether she was feeding correctly, whether the house was clean and in order. Beth was exhausted and before long she didn't even want to leave the house, leaving her more and more isolated.

The guilt that accompanied her mental torment was intolerable. She was told that she should be feeling on top of the world, and she saw other mothers in the street seemingly happy and content. Her mother-in-law told her to just be thankful that she had a healthy baby and commented that women had it much harder back in *her* day. Beth felt so embarrassed about feeling unwell in her mind, especially because she had really did have an easy life, and the shame led to deeper depression. Eventually, after watching her state worsen, her husband took her to their local doctor.

The medical appointment was highly uncomfortable for Beth and she felt as if she was being treated like a crazy person. Her doctor explained that medication was the recommended pathway to recovery and that he would write her a prescription; her husband agreed that it was the best way forward. Beth argued and argued that she wanted to try other strategies first and that she needed some more help from her husband with the baby and some more sleep to just feel human again. She felt completely shut down by both her doctor and her husband as they told her that she wasn't in any fit state to make those kinds of decisions.

I have experienced stigma many times and it is always demoralising. Like Beth, I've had someone dictate what I must do and take to regain mental stability, and have endured questions regarding my ability to make sound decisions, all adding to feelings of failure and shame.

Stigma is a terrible thing. Unfortunately, media has painted a picture where most violent criminal offenders are mentally ill. This may be accurate, but no context is given to the spectrum involved in mental illness. I argue that there is a spectrum for all illness of the mind, and those who are prone to violent criminal acts due to pathology are at the pointy end of the spectrum. Few travel there, and many do so with the help of illicit drugs.

In the past I have grappled with embarrassment, and been scared out of my mind when contemplating divulging my mental-health challenges to more than a couple of key people (clearly I have moved beyond that in writing this book). Yet ask me about the time I fractured my ankle, or caught chickenpox from my kids in my late twenties and I'll go into great detail about how I stayed in bed for a week and spent days bathing in vibrant red anti-itching lotion. Even now it's far more acceptable to speak about physical ailments than mental.

~

Stigma: a mark of disgrace associated with a particular circumstance, quality, or person.

Synonyms: shame, disgrace, dishonour.

Independent of severe mental illness, there are a number of potential factors that can prevent us from feeling well in our mind: stress, lack of social support, loneliness, poor gut health, poor dietary choices, hormone imbalance, inflammation, childhood trauma, shame, rumination, betrayal of trust, sleep disturbances, screen time, alcohol abuse, unnoticed head injury, thyroid disturbances.[9] I would bet that each and every one of us has experienced at least one (if not more) of these factors.

We may go to our doctor because we feel discomfort in our mind, and at our consultation our doctor might consider our set of symptoms and diagnose a disorder. It's not that simple, as we see through Beth's story. Beth knew what she needed. She needed support and help with her newborn. Instead she had her power taken from her.

And so, many factors can contribute to an unwell mind and can lead to symptoms listed in the Diagnostic and Statistical Manual (DSM), used worldwide by clinicians and psychiatrists to diagnose mental illness. The current version DSM 5 has received much criticism in the psychological health arena, with assertions that it will lead to 'massive over diagnosis and harmful over medication'.[10]

The gene-based model embraced in allopathic medicine would have us believe that if we are sick or suffering with a broken mind, we are lumped with that for life; it's in our genes, right? No. We have an element of control over genetic predisposition. We can both prevent and heal.

No such thing as normal

I'm sure we can all think of people who seemingly have it all together? But do they really? Struggle in our mind is part of living, so you can be sure that everyone will struggle internally. To be human is profoundly hard.

Also, we can assume that none of us is unique in terms of what we struggle with, but we do have different ways of showing our struggle. For example, I tend to be stoic in front of others, hiding behind a mask of 'It'll be right' even when nothing feels like it will be right again. Others may call a friend and cry, or seek therapy, or self-soothe in addictions (I am prone to this as well), or hide behind rigid and controlling behaviour. We all have a defensive scaffold so we can hide and withdraw. These are our coping mechanisms.

I have been told by those who haven't lived with me, but are aware of my diagnosis, that I appear so 'normal'. It makes me curious as to what the collective definition of 'normal' is.

I'm absolutely passionate about this: when it comes to mental health, there is no normal. In fact, a study published in 2018, *The Myth of Optimality in Clinical Neuroscience*,[11] by Yale University Psychology Department, debunked the term 'normal'. The authors make an impressive argument, stating that differences and variety in living species (the same species) are far *more* common than uniformity.

The authors conclude that despite popular belief, no universally optimal profile of brain functioning exists. And it gets better when they state: *'we propose that, instead of examining behaviours in isolation, psychiatric illnesses can be best understood through the study of domains of functioning and associated [complex] patterns of variation across distributed brain systems.'*

What this means is that attempting to define a people by their divergence from some model, from a psychiatric perspective, is a really sad way of disempowering that person. How can that person connect with their true self, if their true self is not considered normal?

We may go to a doctor with symptoms of anxiety, and then be assessed in a linear, one-size-fits-all approach, all while the world is expansive and in a perpetual state of flux. This is not to say that if we are suffering we shouldn't seek help from a caring physician, but I would suggest that the care sought should be integrated, as opposed to merely prescriptive.

To clarify: if we are struggling with anxiety we should be assessed on several determinants, rather than adopting a single screening tool. Nutritional status, gut health, environmental factors, exposure to toxins, family relationships and more play a role in our mental wellness; therefore these factors should be considered part of the solution. This is in stark contrast to the current scenario of screening for a diagnosis and being prescribed a suitable pharmaceutical drug.

Does medication give us control?

I have had quite a bumpy ride with medication. Mood stabilisers can have nasty side effects such as drowsiness, thirst and nausea, and taking several pills a day is hard. They aren't magic pills, either. The crests and crashes of swinging moods were still often there, and it was always a constant tweaking: I felt like a lab rat in my own experiment.

Of importance is that I believed that medication was the first line of defence for me — and only that. I didn't believe that it was going to save me. I had to save myself.

We put so much trust in the medical world, while not understanding that the research is also accessible for us. In fact, doctors and psychiatrists are incredibly busy people, saving lives and attending an endless stream of patient needs. Sometimes, we have more time to read up on new tools available to help us heal our mind than they do. Rather than give our health practitioners total control, we need to partner with them.

Please note: I am not suggesting that we all boycott medical advice and take matters into our own hands. Medical practitioners are highly trained professionals with a wealth of knowledge. I am only suggesting that you be proactive with your approach to your journey to mental wellness.

Denise's story

Denise had a really bad year. A close friend died suddenly, she was retrenched from her job, and a number of large expenses had engulfed her savings. Small problems that previously wouldn't have bothered her became monumental. Her newly unemployed status meant that she had more time on her hands, but nothing of substance to focus on. She soon slipped into a depressed state. Motivation to get out of bed in the morning evaporated, evenings were spent with several glasses of wine, days were spent bathing in self-loathing.

Feeling like she was on a downward spiral into despair, Denise booked an appointment with her doctor. At his advice she began taking antidepressants, and started to feel better immediately. The fog lifted, and a little motivation returned, but she was still grieving for her friend, unemployed and anxious. She also felt a level of emotional disconnection and fatigue, and her sex drive vanished.

After six months of medicating, Denise decided she wanted to stop. She felt that the medication was dulling her emotions, that she had lost the richness of experiencing life's ups and downs. She weaned herself off the medication and what followed was a dreadful couple of months. It was so difficult that she almost gave up and recommenced medication.

In fact, she felt worse than when she had started the medication. The withdrawal from this type of medication is called 'discontinuation syndrome' and can manifest as irritability, insomnia, headaches, flu-like symptoms, nausea and the return of depressive symptoms.[12]

It would appear that although antidepressants have a place, and can help in extreme cases, for most of us they assist us to simply function, which is miles away from thriving. To thrive means that we live with a sense of meaning and gratitude and flow through the full spectrum of moods and feelings.

Denise struggled immensely and so sought advice from a holistic medical practitioner. She was advised to cut her pills in half for four weeks, and then into quarters for the remainder of her supply. Denise started to walk for 30 minutes daily and was vigilant in keeping a regular bed time. She started a supplement regime under her health practitioner's care and booked a consultation with a nutritionist.

Even after Denise had weaned completely off medication it was still a bumpy ride for a time. She felt emotionally fragile since having her emotions blunted by the medication, and because she hadn't worked through the grief leading up to the diagnosis she was feeling very low. It took a couple of months for the emotional roller-coaster to subside: when it did, Denise reclaimed her power. She reminded herself that she had the inner strength to overcome; that her suffering was just a season. She was proud that she found light inside herself even when she was drowning in darkness.

The downside of medication

If current treatment for mental illness was really effective, vast numbers of people would report rates of remission. This isn't the case. As mentioned (see page 20), we are treating a neurotransmitter imbalance in the mind, and yet, for depression at least, the link between symptoms and low levels of the chemical serotonin has been challenged, and is now believed untenable.[13] SSRIs are still commonly prescribed because we want a nice easy fix to our dis-ease.* However, unfortunately, these drugs have a plethora of side effects and, in most cases, are really difficult to wean off. In fact, we are often led to believe that these medications are a lifelong commitment; therefore we aren't supposed to come off them.

The majority of studies investigating the effectiveness of antidepressants are funded by pharmaceutical companies, and often the trials last only eight weeks. Although it may be considered unnecessary to conduct longer trials, the long-term outcomes of these drugs should be evaluated. In regards to the efficiency of these medications, criticism has been directed at the short duration of eight-week studies.[14]

Robert Whitaker,[15] a journalist and author who compiles published data and reviews on psychiatry and antidepressants, focuses on risk versus benefit in regards to psychotropic medication.

---

*Dis-ease: a trendy, and often criticised, way of pointing out that most disease comes from a lack of ease.

Whitaker thoughtfully poses the question: do those who get well on antidepressants stay well? It is an important question.

He discusses the work of John Rush, a prominent psychiatrist at the University of Texas Southwestern, and a study conducted in 2004 of the effectiveness of antidepressants in 118 real-world patients.[16] Whitaker highlights that in this study 13 percent of people on antidepressants were in remission at the end of the year, and only 5 percent had a sustained remission during the following year. Whitaker discusses research conducted by Michael Posternak, a psychiatrist at Brown University, in 2006 looking at one-year remission rates for unmedicated patients.[17] Posternak identified 84 patients enrolled in the NIMH STAR*D trial — the largest antidepressant trial conducted. He recruited those who, after recovering from an initial bout of depression, subsequently relapsed but did not go back on an antidepressant.

He tracked the remission rate of these patients over time and reported that 23 percent had recovered by the end of the first month; 67 percent at the end of six months, and 85 percent at the end of one year. What this means is that 85 percent of unmedicated participants had full remission of depressive symptoms after one year. Unmedicated!

Kelly Brogan MD — who has adopted the title 'renegade' psychiatrist — has worked tirelessly to help her patients get off medication and dig into the root of their mental-health issues. Receiving much criticism along the way, Dr Brogan is vocal and committed. Recently she published an article discussing the belief that medication should be the first port of call to heal our mind.[18] She brings to light a meta-analysis conducted by both Dr Irving Kirsch, Associate Director of the Program in Placebo Studies and a lecturer in medicine at the Harvard Medical School,[19] and Dr JC Fournier, Assistant Professor of Psychiatry, University of Pittsburgh School of Medicine,[20] which highlights a potent placebo effect in all but the most severe cases of depression.

This means that those who were allocated to a placebo pill, rather than an antidepressant, improved significantly. Not so with those suffering severe depression, however — the benefit reported in these patients may have been observed due to a rating scale referring to side effects such as sedation, or activation (improved sleep or energy). These are likely to be unrelated to a primary pharmacologic action of serotonin production. This does not mean that we are to entirely disregard medication in relation to mental illness, but it does highlight the need for mindful consideration.

Doctors are very quick to prescribe medication — and this isn't only confined to psychotropic medication. Antibiotics are also over-prescribed[21] and will lead to poor gut health, which in turn increases risk of anxiety, depression and more. Medication is a tool and can work wonders for some, but for others different tools are more effective. In regards to antidepressant use, long-term studies on efficiency and safety are lacking. Also there are suggestions that depression is often over-diagnosed, as well as overtreated.[22]

There have been occasions when avoiding my regular doctor (yes, that's a thing), I would visit another and go home with antidepressant drugs, minus mood stabilisers. Antidepressants are the worst type of drug for a bipolar patient such as me because they exacerbate mania. The irritable anger was unbearable and I would scream and cry all day until I had worn myself out. Physically I was spent but my mind kept racing. I would then stop taking medication and sink into worse depression.

You may feel you have an unwell mind, or you may feel anxious, or stressed, apathetic or just plain sad. No matter what your state, there are many tools to help you feel better.

There may be another way

Doctors generally don't ask in a consultation how many serves of oily fish you consume, or whether you take magnesium supplements, or a probiotic. Most doctors rarely prescribe nutrition and lifestyle changes for a patient who presents with an unwell mind — and yet that is often exactly what is needed.

From another perspective, there is strong evidence linking poor nutrition and lifestyle choices with mental illness, so we cannot expect our doctor to undo twenty or so years of damage inflicted by our poor health practices. If we spend a decade or two neglecting our health, we will suffer consequences — and our medical practitioners want to help us, and so prescribe medication.

The saying 'Diagnose and adios' depicts this perfectly. We go in with a problem and leave with a prescription. My intention is not to suggest that medication should never be considered — sometimes it is necessary. My intention is to provide other avenues you can explore. There is no such thing as a quick fix to truly heal our mental and emotional health; it is solely *our* responsibility to do the work, and we must soak up all the knowledge we can.

Although, technically, I have a diagnosis that suggests that my brain is broken, I believe that had I been taught how to take care of my mind from a young age, just like I was taught to care for my body, I may never have received that diagnosis.

Humans are complex creatures and somewhere along the way we have given up ownership of the health of our mind and body. A theme I will visit often through this book is ownership. We must own our mind, whatever state it is currently in, and take back control.

CHAPTER 2:

Mindset

'Challenges are what make life interesting.
Overcoming them is what makes life meaningful.'

Joshua J Marine

There are several mindsets that we adopt through life. And there are several reasons one person may adopt a particular mindset, and someone else another. I have often questioned why I developed the drive to heal my mind while others who have been diagnosed with the same pathology wind up homeless, unemployed and/ or on medication for life. It's not because I am better, smarter or luckier. It is simply that I believed that my mind could be healed.

What are some of the driving forces that fuel the mindset we adopt? It's a complicated topic because humans are complex creatures, but let's delve into it anyway.

~

Avoidance mentality doesn't work

Although the brain is a complex and awesome machine, it still has primitive wiring designed for three things: to seek pleasure, to preserve energy and to avoid pain. These innate behaviours served our survival in Paleolithic and Neolithic times, driving humans to seek pleasure through companionship, sex and procreation. The pleasure drive facilitated our survival as a species. Additionally, we sought out high-energy foods, and fell into hibernation to conserve energy for survival. We did our utmost to avoid pain, because pain can kill. This is what got us here.

We are still seeking pleasure, but now it is in abundance. That, in itself, is creating a precarious environment in our mind. For most people in developed countries, food is plentiful, access to entertainment is easy, and numbing agents such as alcohol and drugs are readily available.

We don't want to feel uncomfortable, yet we must be able to feel discomfort and be able to sit with it. Attempts to avoid it are a recipe for disaster because the avoidance mentality results in mental pain, and delays healing. Back in the day we had to avoid pain to survive, but now we avoid discomfort because it feels bad.

Control

Before I took control of my mental wellbeing, I felt like a failure most of the time. The not-so-funny aspect of being diagnosed with a mental illness is that although friends and family are aware of a 'pathology', they still expect normal behaviour, and if we don't manage to deliver, a feeling of defeat sets in. Because some friends and family would comment that I was overly emotional, reactive, impulsive and just too much, I would try with all my might to hide those traits. Then, when I failed, I would spiral. I had dreams of being calm, logical and wise: in reality I was on the edge of a cliff ready to topple at any time.

When my children were babies I developed OCD. Perhaps it was always there, but it manifested noticeably after I had kids. I would dust the bookshelves, blinds, light fittings, furniture — whatever I could reach — at least 100 times each day. No, I'm not exaggerating. I remember having a friend over for lunch and getting the dust buster out to suck up the crumbs she left on the table after feeding her a tantalizing gourmet sandwich: while she was still sitting at the table … eating the sandwich!

We moved as a young family every six to twelve months (I got bored easily). I loved to pack up the house quickly, move, then scrub everything clean and unpack in new surroundings.

In addition to the dust-free (and different) house, security was paramount for me. Each night I would check each and every window and door at least a dozen times. It was exhausting. I would then check my sleeping babies countless times. The rituals and routines made me feel safe and I was quite sure if I neglected them that calamity would ensue.

Also, I felt an enormous sense of responsibility. Like if I didn't appear okay, then everything would fall apart. I had to be 'on' all the time; to be there for friends and family whenever they needed anything; to fix the problems of the world; to be the best that I could be. It's a delusion of control. I believed I had control over everything (just not my emotional outbursts). I would hold myself responsible for everything that went wrong and carried the weight of the world on my shoulders.

I also had an exaggerated view of my power over others. If I didn't fix everyone else's problems, right every wrong, or meet every need, the world would fall apart. I felt guilt when I couldn't patch up the wounds of others, and if something went wrong I blamed myself. I was a people pleaser and falsely believed that I was more important than I am. The truth is that others manage just fine without me and that the world will not fall apart if I'm not busy fixing everything.

I have had to work hard to overcome this mindset, and I'm sure that I still have an inner control freak that rears her head far too often. But I see it for what it is: it is fear.

We are hardwired to be fearful. The human psyche is brilliantly and beautifully protective, but at the same time this protective mechanism can be burdensome and detrimental. Back when we were cavemen doing our cavemen stuff, paying attention to the bad things was a lifesaver. Being fearful kept us on our toes and alive. Those attuned to dangerous situations lived to tell the tale, while happy-go-lucky souls were gobbled up by wild beasts. So, it paid off to be suspicious and wary, because those who were on alert all the time survived the perils of the day.

The human brain dislikes uncertainty; hence, we strive to control certain aspects of our life. This can become dysregulated, as in my case. My need to control my environment and my misplaced sense of power to impact the lives of others was driven by fear. Fear that my world would fall apart if I didn't have control. Fear of failure, fear of exclusion, fear of uncertainty.

On the other end of a spectrum of control are those who believe that they have little or no control, and that something or someone else controls what happens to them. For example, they often think things like, 'I can't lose weight because my parents always fed me too much as a child,' or 'I can't change my mindset because I have too much stress in my life,' or 'I'm too old and no one will want me.' This kind of thinking takes away power and leaves us helpless, and is also driven by fear. The sense of responsibility that accompanies control can be scary: sometimes it's easier to blame circumstances or others, rather than assume responsibility ourselves.

When we believe that we are responsible for everyone else, a pattern of guilt and poor self-esteem follows, which can develop into shame. When we believe that we have no control over anything, we don't take action, and action is necessary to change our circumstances. Action may not lead to instant results, but without action you can be sure your mental health and wellbeing won't reach full potential.

Another mindset that contributes to an unwell mind is the belief that we are on this beautiful planet to simply live a happy existence.

But we are meant to be happy!

We have all been sold the idea that bad things shouldn't happen, and that when they do occur they disrupt the journey to a much-coveted state of constant happiness. *No.* Happiness will never be a constant state, bad things do happen often, and a number of evolutionary and learned facets of human behaviour mean there will always be struggle within.

In the past we were rarely taught how to achieve optimal emotional health, which is unfortunate, because our emotions drive everything. This is changing thankfully as schools are implementing wellbeing programs into the curriculum. However, we still often adhere to the notion that external factors make us happy or sad, that other people have the power to hurt our feelings, that other things *cause* our feelings. This is just not true. Our thoughts cause our feelings. The good news is that our thoughts are one thing we *do* have control over.

When we cultivate the belief that external influences have control over how we feel, we adopt the mantra:

If only our circumstances changed …

If only that person loved me more …

If only we had more money …

We would feel happy.

We then look out into the world through the lens of social media or advertising, and we see photoshopped, happy, perfect poses. Perfect bodies. Faultless families. So, we feel that everyone else is happy and living perfect lives, and therefore we are not normal: there must be something wrong with us.

Because we are meant to be happy, damn it!

Anxiety often follows because we aren't *doing* enough to obtain that perfect, happy life. And, because that feels uncomfortable, we self-medicate with buffers (food, alcohol, drugs, porn, shopping) to ease the pain of not being normal or happy. We don't talk to our friends or colleagues about the angst that we feel. Instead we believe we need to push it down, because they aren't talking about it either.

We strive to numb pain because pain is uncomfortable; but attempts to avoid pain delay healing. Most times psychological pain is transitory, so if we move through it at the time of its genesis we can heal it then and there. I know— easier said than done.

The false premise that we can attain long-term happiness or satisfaction in an unsatisfactory world is just damaging. *Dukkha*, an important Buddhist term, is often explained as 'life being filled with suffering', but the correct translation is 'unsatisfactory' or 'unsatisfying'. Life is unsatisfying most of the time, which may be related to that existential angst that most of us experience at some point. This makes sense because most of the things that provide us with satisfaction pass away. You may reach the goal, or get the 'thing' ... but it's not permanent, or the feeling associated is only temporary. You can only say, 'I did it, I did it,' and celebrate after you reach your goal for so long before it gets weird. So, then you move on. Everything dissipates, even the most pleasant of experiences. Comfort does not last, even when you are at your most comfortable; the feeling associated will leave and you will then search for more comfort.

On the plus side, the same can be said for unpleasant experiences. Everything passes, even the bad. Discomfort and pain work the same way: the feeling leaves you eventually.

So, happiness is transient. And do you agree: if we were happy all the time we would be *so* boring? A sense of meaning is what fills us up.

A study published in the *Proceedings of the National Academy of Sciences* in 2013 reported that people who are happy but lack meaning in their lives show the same gene expression patterns as those whose immune system is struggling to fight off bacterial infections.[23] In other words, they are inflamed. If this continues in a prolonged state it can increase the risk of major illnesses such as cancer and heart disease, because the body is in a constant state of inflammation. Now, this sounds like being happy is bad for us. No, not quite. According to the researchers, the problem isn't with being happy but that self-perception of meaningfulness is outweighed by happiness.

And unfortunately this is fairly common. People with high happiness scores and low meaningfulness scores accounted for 75 percent of the study's participants. Only 25 percent actually had more meaning in their lives than happiness.

Friedrich Nietzsche[24] was a nineteenth-century German philosopher who believed we really don't desire happiness. Rather, he proposed that we need struggle, because that's where we find meaning, and meaning is what makes us happy.

Nietzsche proposed that man needs to believe that life has a meaning or purpose, simply because he suffers so deeply and therefore wants to be assured that he suffers for a reason. And this very belief that life has meaning and purpose makes us happy. Happiness is merely a by-product, according to Nietzsche (supported by many other philosophers).[25] 'Joy accompanies, joy does not move,' he stated. A person renovating their house isn't doing so because it makes them happy (it's more likely to cause them pain), but the joy felt when it is completed is an awesome bonus.

I'll say it again: we are complex creatures who have many hurdles to overcome in the journey to feel the best that we can.

CHAPTER 3:

The Stories We Cling To

'You only have control over three things in your life — the thoughts you think, the images you visualize, and the actions you take.'

Jack Canfield

The stories we recite to ourselves define us. These stories can become one of the hurdles to overcome on our way to mental wellness. We create a whole life around beliefs that were shaped in us during the first seven years of life. A common narrative of my life was that I am not enough; I'm guessing that's not uncommon.

When I was around seven years old my step-sister came to live with us. She was fourteen, super cool and not particularly nice to me, but I thought she was a rock star. I had the biggest crush on the boy who lived across the road (we had practised kissing a few times — I started young). I thought that he loved me — until I saw him look at my step-sister. Suddenly he wanted her to play Sandy opposite his Danny in our rendition of *Grease*. I had been cast aside for an older, cuter, cooler girl.

Seven years later, my first boyfriend (my ex-husband) also dumped me for an older, cuter, cooler woman. That is the story I have proclaimed to myself in romantic relationships: I'm replaceable and not enough — and it produces fear, which has historically manifested as anger, jealousy, anxiety and other unsociable behaviours.

Now, this is just one example: there are many! These stories keep us locked in prisons of isolation and ego.

When I was lecturing, occasionally students would leave my class early, and every time this happened I went to the familiar, 'I am not enough … I am not a good enough teacher to hold their attention … I said something stupid … I am boring, my lectures are not as interesting as their other classes,' et cetera. This is because I was familiar with telling myself this story, and it reinforced what I felt in younger years: I am not enough.

I could have just thought, 'Those lazy little sods are skipping out on half a lecture!' Or I could have considered alternatives: maybe they had an appointment, perhaps they were hungover and needed a Panadol, or maybe they wanted to study for an upcoming test, or go to the beach.

I had to get to a place where I understood that I was not born with a tag on my back reading 'easily replaced', or 'not enough'. Just as none of us is born with a tag stating, 'I don't have enough, I'm not capable enough, I don't deserve, I don't have time, I can't leave, I can't …'

It's not reality, it's only a story.

We all have them — stories that we tell ourselves, often without even realizing we are doing it. Then we take that narrative and make it our truth. The stories may be negative, or even delusional such as, 'If I just ignore it, the problem will go away.' Rather than taking a victim stance, why don't we rewrite the story and start to look at our past from a different angle? Use the questions below to think about your own stories and how they impact your life today.

The stories we tell

Reflect on stories you created from negative experiences when young. Think of a time you felt like you weren't good enough, had enough, or similar, and write it down.

When in recent years have you recreated that feeling?

Take the story you have recalled above and now retell it. For example, you weren't invited to Tom's birthday party in high school. You felt you weren't popular enough. Recently you weren't included on the invitation list for a corporate lunch, so you revisited the feeling of not being liked and wallowed in self-pity. Now retell the story as 'I didn't make much effort with Tom at school and didn't really have much in common with that crowd. The people I mix with now all include me most of the time. I guess it was an oversight that I wasn't on the invitation list.'

Embrace the fact that those stories are inaccurate. Have you ever been so sure that someone disliked you because they didn't seem warm on your first meeting, only to become besties with them months later, learning that they felt intimidated by you at that first meeting?

If you ever find yourself saying to yourself (not out loud — that would be crazy), 'I can't draw to save myself: I was always really bad at art in school,' or 'I can't possibly learn ballroom dancing, I have always had two left feet,' or 'I am the way I am, due to the trauma I experienced growing up,' or 'I'm too old, too fat, too uptight, too young, too loud, too timid, too scared, too unfit, too unco-ordinated, too unintelligent, too … for that,' stop and remind yourself that it's only a story that you carry, possibly due to past experience and beliefs, or primitive fear of danger. The stories are *not* true.

~

Feed the right wolf

An old Cherokee was teaching his grandson about life.

'A fight is going on inside me,' he said to the boy. 'It is a terrible fight and it is between two wolves. One is evil — he is anger, envy, sorrow, regret, greed, arrogance, self-pity, guilt, resentment, inferiority, lies, false pride, superiority and ego.'

He continued, 'The other is good — he is joy, peace, love, hope, serenity, humility, kindness, benevolence, empathy, generosity, truth, compassion and faith. The same fight is going on inside you — and inside every other person, too.'

The grandson thought about it for a minute and then asked his grandfather: 'Which wolf will win?'

The old Cherokee simply replied, 'The one you feed.'

It takes no effort to feed the first wolf. The second wolf is trickier: it takes time and effort and often goes against what we naturally desire to do. However, if we persevere and focus more on feeding the second wolf, we will suffer less in the long term. The wolf we choose to feed also defines the stories we allow to grow inside us.

Rejection

A sturdy road block to mental wellness is rejection. Rejection is a fear that most humans perpetually live with, and we have all been rejected in one way or another. Perhaps you can relate to the following example?

Kira had a terrible relationship with her father. He was a hard, critical man who didn't have anything positive to say to either her or her brother. For example, when she was six years old she made him a birthday card at school and proudly put it on his bedside table. She waited and waited, filled with hope that he would see the card and be filled with love for his neglected daughter. Minutes ticked over into hours, and hours into days and there was no mention of the card.

Time went by and Kira grew, eventually moved out and married. The relationship with her father remained fractured and she carried those early wounds through adolescence and then adulthood. Kira managed to function well despite the emotional pain she carried, and no one would have suspected that she had felt so utterly unloved by her father.

One day after a particularly tough day at work, Kira's husband came home, tired and irritable. He sat in front of the TV and didn't say a word to Kira. She had spent an hour in the kitchen cooking his favourite meal — and she hated cooking. He had just grumbled that he wasn't hungry and went to bed.

For someone else, this might have inflicted a small graze that healed quickly after apologies and explanations were dispensed regarding his horrible mood. But for Kira, this was a large cut in her already open and festering wound, and feelings of safety within her marriage were dealt a blow. She had, in earlier years, developed a habit of putting up walls anytime she was at risk of being rejected or hurt. She did this to avoid the childhood pain that she had suffered. She would swallow the hurt rather than confront it, and just pull away a little more. The rejection from her father had shadowed her through life and the pain now permeated her marriage.

Kira had to reach a place where she could reflect on her father's behaviour as his problem — not hers. Her father had demons that had been passed down from his father and had nothing to do with Kira and her value. When she realised that the feeling of safety in her marriage had been compromised, she sought help.

Like most of us, Kira had some work to do, such as catching her assumptions before they settled in. She did this by reflecting, asking, 'Is there any proof I am being rejected in this situation?' She then asked what other possible assumptions could be made in place of rejection. She started to analyse her emotions rather than respond or shut down. This helped significantly.

Another tool Kira adopted when feeling rejection was to allow herself to dwell on the emotions and pain just briefly. Then she would move on to notice the thoughts that accompany the feelings.

For example, she would think, 'I'm having the thought that I am not loved by my husband as he doesn't want to spend time with me right now, but it's just a thought, how do I know it's true?'

My biological father walked away after meeting me once: just after I was born. I have only recently learned that he was married to another woman at the time (my mum wasn't aware of what a busy man he was) and his wife was pregnant with my half-sister. For decades I had assumed that I wasn't enough for him to want to be part of my life.

Because my fear of rejection had grown so strong based on that belief, I would rush to end relationships, and even friendships, or push others away if I so much as got an inkling that they were withdrawing first. My father did not leave because I wasn't enough: he left because he didn't want to bring shame on himself, so he took the easy way out. It had nothing at all to do with me and I had been telling myself an inaccurate story for nearly 40 years.

We all experience feelings of rejection at some point. Even the best rock band in the world (the best according to me), U2, received a rejection letter from RSO records. And, sometimes we are too sensitive to rejection and don't consider alternative reasons for the perceived snub.

Our fear of rejection has been suggested to arise from our primitive brain, which wasn't too flash at reflection and self-analysis. Humans are social creatures, and in hunter–gatherer days we used to coexist with bands of 25–40 tribe mates. If our social group decided we weren't part of the 'cool' crowd, then we were kicked out into the cold, dangerous night alone. So, if we were rejected from our tribe it literally meant death because we couldn't survive on our own. So, we are hardwired to take things personally and remain alert for signs of rejection.

The way we are wired

Many regions of our brain are buried in the most primordial parts of our mind and are thought to be among the first to develop in primitive humans. The limbic system is important because it houses the amygdala (see Figure 2 on page 71), which plays a role in attaching emotion to events and memories,[26] and may create fear. When the amygdala senses that you are facing a threat, it sends out nerve impulses to another part of the brain: the hypothalamus. The hypothalamus activates the pituitary gland and the pituitary gland activates the adrenal gland. The adrenal gland secretes stress hormones adrenaline, noradrenaline and cortisol, and these trigger the fight-or-flight response.

Some trivia

Several studies involving rats have used deep lesioning (a procedure where a thin wire is inserted into the brain to remove or terminate a part of the brain) to remove the amygdala. After the removal of the amygdala, the rats were reported to not fear anything, even cats.

Also, recent research out of the University of Pennsylvania reported a link between the structure of a person's brain and a propensity towards risk-taking.[27] There are a number of different factors involved in a person's tendency to avoid or take risks: this study focused on the brain regions engaged in risk taking — the amygdala, and the medial prefrontal cortex, which aids with decision making and long-term memory. The study involved participants in a gambling scenario, and looked at how willing individuals were to accept the risk of getting nothing for the chance of getting a higher amount of money. One hundred and eight participants took part in the study and had to choose between a set financial gain of twenty dollars, or a larger risky reward that varied from trial to trial, and may have resulted in no win at all.

Magnetic Resonance Imaging and Diffusion Tensor Imaging tools were used to measure the size of the amygdala and the volume of grey and white matter in the amygdala before testing and then the data was compared to risk-taking behaviour during the test. They also measured the connectedness between the amygdala and medial prefrontal cortex. It was concluded that individuals with a larger amygdala and greater connectiveness displayed a higher tolerance for risk taking.

~

The amygdala in our primitive brain was super important in Paleolithic times because it helped us remember dangers and where they lay.[28] These days it helps us to remember the emotions attached to certain scenarios occurring throughout our life. Therefore, some stories we hold onto evolve from the primitive brain. Perhaps we got laughed at while singing at school assembly; 30 years later we are self-conscious anytime we get caught belting out Abba's 'Dancing Queen' while cooking dinner (or is that just me?).

Also interesting with regard to the amygdala is that this area of the brain is linked to impulsivity, and may influence decision making. I'll discuss that in more detail soon.

So, most of the stories we cling to and the fears that walk with us are a fundamental and deeply wired reaction to protect us from threat and harm. We all fear being demeaned or cut off from others and we put up illusionary scaffolding to protect ourselves. For a well mind, we need to tear it all down.

CHAPTER 4:

A Paradox

'The world as we created it is a process of our thinking.
It cannot be changed without changing our thinking.'

Albert Einstein

We want to be happy but we give more weight to the negative: go figure!

My stepchildren like to remind me of the time I ran out of petrol. I had had such a busy week, because we were moving house. Admittedly, I sometimes let the needle on the fuel gauge slip below the quarter-full mark, but as soon as I notice I go and fill up. But that week I was flustered and tired and so I didn't even notice when the 'danger' light had come on. And there we were: empty on the side of the road on a hot February day. And I still hear about it two years on. What if I flipped it? What if I asked my stepkids, 'Well, how many times have I filled up the car so we *didn't* run out of petrol?' I am sure they couldn't care less about that, understandably.

We care about negative occurrences in life, rather than the positive. Changing our mindset is not easy when we are more inclined to focus on the negative and be reactive to adverse situations. The negative attracts our attention because we are wired for self-protection, and then we react from emotion rather than intellect.

Julia Roberts' character Vivian, in the movie *Pretty Woman*, sums up: 'The bad stuff is easier to believe. You ever notice that?' This is correct in most cases: bad is stronger than good, because the bad takes longer to process than the good, and so stays present with us for longer, and is therefore easier to believe.

A study conducted at Harvard Business School by Teresa M Amabile, Professor at Harvard Business School, and Steven J Kramer, psychologist and researcher, aimed to tease out the events that make or break a working day for over 200 professional employees. One focus of the study was what effect a setback had on the whole working day. Over four months participants worked on different projects and kept a daily journal.[29] The researchers then analysed over 12,000 diary entries looking at the effects of both positive and negative events occurring during the employees' day-to-day activities.

This research highlighted that the negative effect of a setback really screwed up the rest of the working day. Any bad thing that occurred in the employee's day, which decreased their progress, affected their happiness more than twice the rate at which a positive event did. Negative events are more powerful than positive. We lean into the negative, which has many implications for our emotional wellbeing.

Alison Ledgerwood[30]—social psychologist and professor from University of California, Davis — tested the hypothesis that humans find it harder to travel from a negative situation, or loss, to a positive situation or gain. Ledgerwood's research included a study in which participants were asked to imagine that an outbreak of a disease had occurred and 600 lives were at stake. In one group, participants were asked to calculate: if 100 lives were saved, how many were lost? The other group had to calculate the lives lost, if 100 lives were saved. The answer for both is of course 500. However, the group that had to calculate losses to gains (the second group), took much longer to calculate than the group that had to figure out the gains to losses.

The researchers concluded that this, in addition to similar studies, shows that once we think of something as a loss it takes work to change it to a gain.[31] We have to *work* to see the upside — it does not come naturally. We will discuss this 'work' later in the book.

False perceptions

We know that our prehistoric brain still rules the roost when it comes to seeking pleasure and avoiding pain, and that this same pathway keeps us fearful and negative, so we are on high alert for danger.

A recent study asked participants if they felt the world was getting better: because apparently, according to key measures of human material wellbeing, it is.[32] The average result was pessimistic to say the least. Although the world is getting better, we generally focus on the bad, and we don't see much hope for the future.

Authors Sam Brinson[33] and Mark Manson[34] expound a separate study, which reveals why this may be the case. It would appear that humans are destined to see problems where there are none, based on past experience.[35] Researchers showed non-colour-blind participants a series of 1000 dots ranging from very blue to purple, and asked them to judge whether each dot was blue. All was well for the first 200 trials where the participants were seeing equal numbers of blue and purple dots, until the scientists decreased the number of blue dots gradually. Well, the human mind couldn't cope, and so the interpretation of the colour blue changed, and participants included the purple dots into the category of blue. This was after being warned, and also paid, for responding to repeated colours the same way at the end of the study as they did at the beginning of the study.

I have been guilty of creating a reality based on past events — I have also been on the receiving end.

After reading so far you, may have gained some insight into my past propensity for aggressive, reactive and irrational behaviour. However, I am now in a place where my nervous system is calm, I can think before reacting, and often exhibit control in even the most stressful situations. Recently there was a family debacle involving yours truly. It was ugly, and upsetting. The other person involved (who has plenty of experience with my pathology), accused me of being aggressive and reactive. However, there was another who witnessed the whole horrid event (with equal experience of my past behaviour). They claimed that I was surprisingly calm, reasonable and restrained (fist pumping all around).

So, it would seem in this case, the imagined behaviour in the heat of an argument was similar to the blue dots disappearing (my past irrational behaviour), and my current calm disposition (the purple dots) being perceived as blue (irrational). Anything I had said or done in that situation would be perceived as unreasonable, based on my past behaviour.

I'm sure we are all guilty of false perceptions at times.

We look for the bad

In the same experiment, participants were shown a large number of mean, menacing faces on the screen, along with some friendly and neutral faces. Just like the blue dots, the mean faces gradually disappeared, after which, participants began to rate the neutral, and even friendly faces as menacing. A similar pattern followed in the third part of the study, when separating unethical research proposals from ethical ones.

We are outwitted so easily! As suggested, and according to the researchers, our brain doesn't make decisions based on reality, rather on prior events or stimuli. And just like the participants in this study demonstrated, we often change our definition of 'what is' to match 'what has been'. Our mind recalibrates its perceptions, based on past experience. The outcome of this study raises the question: How can we ever be sure that we see things as they really are?

If humans are wired like this, then any time a problem is solved we may expand the definition of the problem to include new problems (think purple dots being perceived as blue). Just as we view the world as getting worse, as opposed to better, we are inclined to do this in our own personal world. And that is certainly going to impact the health and wellbeing of our mind.

Let's face it, it has never been the job of our brain to allow us to skip through life happy and content — it was designed to see danger everywhere. Thanks to our brain we were scared enough of the lion in prehistoric times to run as fast as we could. Those caught swanning around, assessing the merits of a 'positive' approach to the situation, soon became lunch.

Not all is lost. At least ten percent of the modern human genome has changed over the past 50,000 years,[36] and our prefrontal cortex has developed considerably, allowing us advanced abilities to plan and reason. We now have better executive functioning and can plan for the future, rather than living in the past. We can consider a multiple range of ideas simultaneously, and develop many problem-solving strategies. Therefore, we can reflect on our primitive hardwiring and find solutions to overcome.

Evolutionary importance of depression

How far back can we trace anxiety, malaise and depression? Do they perhaps serve a purpose? Just as anxiety and paranoia ensured that we stayed away from the rustling in the bushes — which may have been a wild and ravenous animal — it may well be that symptoms of depression such as fatigue, loss of sex drive, loss of appetite and lack of motivation were birthed in the evolutionary requirement to fight off infections throughout history. These symptoms would ensure the sufferer would lie low, and 'feel low', so that all available resources were poured into keeping the patient alive, and give them time to heal.

These evolutionary tools to keep us alive (yes, even our sugar and fat cravings) are extraordinarily mismatched with the environment in which we live today, and we need to learn to override them.

The symptoms of inflammation that catapulted primitive humans into survival mode to fight the infection are the same observed today. With one exception. We now know that inflammation is not only caused by viral or bacterial pathogens, but can be produced in the body by poor dietary choices, and even stress, leading to chronic inflammation. Consider this for a moment. Studies have shown that mental illness arises from inflammation.[37] And inflammation is caused by a range of factors present in our modern Western civilisation. The 'survival mode', or symptoms to encourage the sufferer to rest when inflammation is present, has not changed. Therefore, symptoms that are listed for depression (fatigue, reduced sex drive, loss of appetite, lack of motivation) may actually be symptoms of chronic systemic inflammation. And because we generally don't have the luxury to stop in our busy lives and resolve the immune response we may find ourselves with chronic depression, chronic anxiety, chronic OCD and more.

More on depression

Depression for me is a sense of feeling hollow. It's like being empty with lights turned down far too low; all you want is for them to be a little brighter, but there is no way to turn them up, so you are stuck in the uncomfortable dimness. When we feel anger, sadness, panic or angst we have somewhere to go: an energy to place somewhere. But in depression, there is no energy to activate anything.

Rather than analysing what deeper factors contribute to our depression, it is more fruitful to treat it as we would the flu. Leave the deep existential questioning to when you are feeling better. If you are unwell, everything looks so bad: when you are depressed the bad is intensified, so it's difficult to really get to the bottom of the cause without magnifying it.

When you have the flu, sleep, nourishment and self-care are important. For me, depression feels like an emotional flu and so I treat it as such without going inward too much. Rest when you can, nourish your body with healthy food, care for yourself as you would do for a sick child, partner or friend.

The traditional approach to achieving mental wellness is to focus on the mind, with medicine to regulate neurotransmitters. We will be focusing on healing the body to build a strong foundation for a well mind.

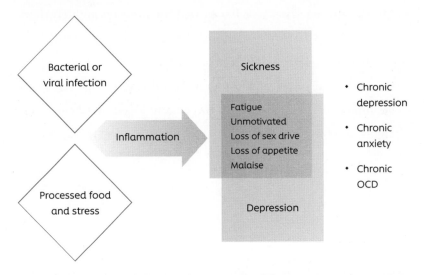

Figure 1. *Bacterial or viral infection caused inflammation in primitive humans resulting in the onset of symptoms to encourage the patient to rest and recover. In modern times we have food and stress, along with other environmental factors that produce inflammation and result in symptoms that are now also associated with depression. When rest is not adequate and inflammation is unresolved, symptoms then progress to the onset of chronic illness of the mind.*

—

So, we know we need to stop drowning in shame and practise self-care; that there are many hurdles to consider on our journey; and that essentially we all struggle.

This next section is where I get excited. After spending many years immersed in nutrition research I want to guide you to make healthy choices to nourish your body to heal your mind. I take a 'food is medicine' approach because if we don't consume enough nutrient-dense foods we become malnourished and sick. Poor nutrition impacts several elements such as our gut microbiome, our immune system, and our physical and mental health and wellbeing. These elements are all related and all important. Trust me: even small changes will have a beneficial effect on how we feel in our mind.

PART 2:

TOOLS TO NOURISH AND PROTECT

CHAPTER 5:

Why We Make
Poor Decisions

*'When inflammation manifests in your body because of
poor health choices, it locks you into the primitive brain,
which is responsible for the impulsive bad decisions.'*

David Perlmutter

There are so many self-help and nutrition books in bookstores; by
and large they are all useless. So, you might say, 'Well, Lisa, why did
you bother to write one?' Great question. What I mean by 'useless'
is, although the information may be correct and worthwhile, unless
we implement the suggestions into our own life, nothing good will
come of it. It will be just another self-help book gathering dust on
your bookshelf.

I am very impulsive, and historically I have made poor decisions. I mostly failed to see the big picture and how my choices would affect me long term. It's a vicious cycle consisting of best intentions, then self-loathing because of another failure. Why do we, even when we know what we should change to feel better, make poor decisions?

There is a reason, and one that can be overcome.

The prefrontal cortex in the brain is influential in decision making, planning for the future, controlling emotions and impulsivity. It's the place we make decisions on what is best for us, for our family, for our environment, and sets us apart from other mammals. Significantly, one-third of our brain consists of prefrontal cortex.

Unfortunately, obesity[38] and inflammation[39] impair the function of the prefrontal cortex. Then, when this important area of the brain is off duty, other areas of the brain can run amok. The main offender is the amygdala, which as we have seen, is connected to the prefrontal cortex.

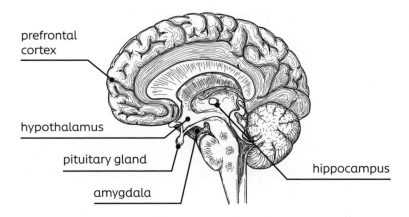

Figure 2. *The prefrontal cortex governs the amygdala. When activity is reduced in the prefrontal cortex due to inflammation, our ability to make long-term decisions for our health and the wellbeing of others is disrupted.*

When the amygdala senses that we are facing a threat, it sends out nerve impulses to another part of the brain: the hypothalamus. The hypothalamus activates the pituitary gland and the pituitary gland activates the adrenal gland. The adrenal gland secretes stress hormones adrenaline, noradrenaline and cortisol, and these trigger the fight-or-flight response.

Dr David Perlmutter and his son Dr Austin Perlmutter, authors of *Brain Wash* have coined the phrase 'disconnection syndrome',[40] which refers to 'the modern disconnection with our DNA; eating foods that the human genome does not recognize'. It is a brilliant and alarming explanation as to why, even when we have access to the right information and know what actions we must take to help our health and wellbeing, we choose the doughnut over the apple.

The authors explain that modern life, inflammatory foods and stress have taken a toll and left a disconnection between the prefrontal cortex and the amygdala. The prefrontal cortex keeps the pesky, fear-producing, risk-taking amygdala in check: when it fails to do so, impulsivity and short-term decisions reign.

There is also a disconnection from the microbiome (rather than nurturing the microbes that promote life and good health, we decimate them with antibacterial sprays and antibiotic use), from the earth, and from each other. Due to disconnection from our prefrontal cortex we make short-term impulsive decisions such as, 'I'm tired, it's late, I'll grab a burger and fries on the way home.' These food choices promote inflammation, which affects our immediate decision-making about food. When we reconnect to our prefrontal cortex we can regain control over our decisions.

CHAPTER 6:

Nourish

'The food you eat can be either the safest and most powerful form of medicine or the slowest form of poison.'

Ann Wigmore

Now … sharing this as a nutrition expert leaves me feeling a little embarrassed and vulnerable.

When I was very mentally unstable I used to drink 2 litres of Coke every day. Throughout my twenties I would wake up each morning and have a cigarette and glass of Coke. I quit Coke and replaced it with a little green can of V (the energy drink) for a while, until I finally gave up sugary drinks (and smoking, thankfully). Other aspects of my diet were considered healthy and I exercised daily, but my nervous system was a mess.

Additionally, I would follow dietary guidelines most of the time. I grew up in the day where it was recommended that we increase our carbohydrate intake to 55–60 percent of total daily energy intake, and that we reduce fat intake. We were told to consume low-fat foods such as skim milk, and replace saturated fats with polyunsaturated fats from inflammatory vegetable oils.

As confessed, my sugar intake was extremely high. Added to that I followed guidelines and ate loads of bread, fruit and cereal products. I cut out saturated fat: I was one of those who hit the gym for a weights workout and then went home to eat egg whites minus the yolk. I counted fat calories whenever I ate, determined to keep fat consumption to under 30 percent of my daily energy intake.

Eating sugar and other refined carbohydrates wreaked havoc on my mind. I was taught to reduce my fat intake and that eating fat would make me fat. Rather than investigating the research myself, I just believed it. Unfortunately, starving my body of essential fatty acids ensured that my mental health suffered, something I have only managed to rectify in recent years. Shifting the way I think about food and understanding that food is information for our body and mind has made such an immeasurable difference to not only my mood but my overall wellbeing.

Scott's story

Scott recalled experiencing anxious thoughts as early as age six. He used to lie in bed at night frozen with fear at every sound, sure that someone was breaking into the house. A nervous child, he regularly experienced butterflies in his stomach and felt jittery and tense. As he grew he became a high achiever, determined to get the best marks on exams and excel in all areas. On the outside he seemed happy and accomplished, but internally he was so tightly wound that a good night's sleep was elusive, and he would spend hours ruminating and obsessing about trivial issues.

Scott had a sweet tooth and ever since he was young had devoured sugary and processed foods. Because he didn't have a weight issue he thought nothing of these dietary practices and would drink sugar-laden drinks, eat sweets, ice-cream and a bag of chips daily.

Scott eventually realized that the anxiety he felt was harder to shift. Heart palpitations, a constant knot in his stomach and cold sweats were now a daily occurrence. He was tired of feeling on constant alert for some unknown threat. His mother booked him into a functional health practitioner recommended by a friend. There, he had a panel of tests: a stool test to check the health of his gut and microbiome, markers of inflammation measured, insulin levels checked, and a full panel ordered to assess thyroid function. Nutrient status including magnesium, B vitamins and vitamin D levels were also assessed.

When the results came back, no one was more surprised than Scott. He was suffering severe dysbiosis in his gut (this refers to an imbalance between good and bad bacteria residing in the gut), and he was deficient in magnesium and vitamin D. He also had high levels of markers of inflammation in his blood samples.

~

Inflammation that occurs after we injure ourselves is referred to as acute inflammation and is important in the healing process. If we injure ourselves and there is swelling, scabbing or redness it's good news because the body is healing itself. But if the immune system ramps up and continues, this is chronic inflammation and is the root of most diseases, including an unwell mind.

Scott walked away from his appointment armed with a nutritional plan to reduce systemic inflammation, a good probiotic to recolonize his gut microbiome, and education on the powerful impact that food and lifestyle changes can have on how we feel in our mind.

Within three months of carefully following his doctor's advice Scott was feeling calm. The knot in his stomach had disappeared and his perspective on life had shifted. He felt energetic, and experienced a sense of peace that he hadn't known was attainable. Weaning himself off processed, sugary foods was incredibly tough, and he faltered a few times before he really hit the road running. Once he had experienced the profound effects on his mind that accompanied nourishing his body and steering clear of junk food, he had no intention of going back.

We *can* own the health of our mind, but it takes work. Many of us know that we don't feel as well as we should, but have been misled by subtle messages in media, from health professionals, from friends and family. The message is that we don't have control. But we *do* have control, and in using the right tools we can all mentally flourish just like Scott.

The current problem

Our ancestors ate loads of fresh vegetables and fruits, wild-caught fish and lean, grass-fed meat. We now eat processed fast food out of boxes, filled with sugar, saturated and trans-fat, colours, preservatives, and fruits and vegetables covered in pesticides and other chemicals.[41]

Progress, being the Agricultural and Industrial revolutions, followed by the globalization of the world food trade, changed our food environment. It is common in Western, affluent countries (and also now in developing countries) to eat carbohydrates that are refined, such as sugar and white flour. Most cereals are made from wheat, and the kind of wheat we now have is far different from what it used to be. We eat processed meat, or grain-fed beef, too much dairy, and too little oily fish. Our food supply is saturated in additives and chemicals.[42]

If you are not moving in wellness circles, you may not even be aware of the evidence demonstrating that this kind of diet is not supporting good mental health (but I'll bet that intuitively you know it's not doing you any favours). In fact, it would seem this changed food supply is the thorn in the side of those of us with predispositions to mind and emotional illness.

S   Standard

A   American (or Western world)

D   Diet

└─→ This way of eating makes us sad!

Jack's story

I first met Jack when he was ten years old. Jack had been diagnosed with high-functioning autism at the age of five. He was presenting with symptoms of anxiety, and his dad stated that he was very slow to respond to instruction. Jack would suffer meltdowns regularly (fits of distress and anger, taking much time to abate). He also suffered from Trichotillomania (pulling out his eyebrows and eyelashes), had a sallow complexion and was quiet and withdrawn.

We looked at Jack's diet. For breakfast he ate cereal and milk, or toast with jam or peanut butter. Lunch was a sandwich made with white bread and ham or other processed meats, chips or cake and an apple and some grapes. Dinner was often pre-packaged food, or grain-fed meat with a few vegetables, pasta, sausages and mash, or hot dogs.

I suggested that significant changes be made to Jack's diet. We started to replace his breakfast of commercial cereal or toast with a smoothie consisting of a banana, some flaxseed, blueberries, spinach, medjool dates, hemp seeds and almond milk. Lunch now consists of sourdough bread with a filling of smoked salmon and cucumber, or avocado, or salad; other lunch choices are an omelette or tuna salad. Dinner is now a big plate of vegetables on most nights with a small portion of lean grass-fed meat, or fish. Snacks include almonds or walnuts, vegetable sticks with hummus, or mixed berries and Greek yoghurt. Sugary treats are kept to a minimum, and water is the only drink he consumes.

Jack is satisfied with his diet, and his favourite foods are a plate of vegetables with cashews, snow peas and haloumi cheese with an avocado sauce on top, or a piece of grilled salmon with vegetables.

Jack has been following the dietary plan for two years now. In that time there have been no reported meltdowns and Jack's eyebrows are growing back, although he does still struggle with Trichotillomania occasionally. Jack's teacher has reported improvements in his schoolwork, and was also surprised by the enthusiasm Jack exhibited at a recent school camp where he took part in all activities and socialised well. Those closest to Jack are happily surprised by his progress.

But what if? What if Jack had continued with poor dietary habits that, let's face it, normally track into adulthood? Would he have still been suffering the meltdowns, the difficulty in focus and trouble with schoolwork? Would he not only pluck out his brows and eyelashes but start on other areas of his body? As a result of poor dietary choices would he suffer further emotional dysregulation that manifests in other illnesses of the mind?

Food and our mind

We can see the terrible effects a poor diet has on the body, with rising obesity rates reported in developed countries. We can't, however, see the insidious effects on the mind. Though an indisputable relationship has been established between diet and brain health,[43] in most cases nutritional therapy is not the first line of attack for mood disorders, or even general malaise. But it should be.

Depression is the leading cause of disability worldwide, and we know that antidepressants are readily dished out. A frightening fact is that of the listed drugs most likely to induce violence, five out of ten are antidepressants,[44] and for some these medications don't work.[45] Although medication is necessary in some cases, what if we can improve our mood without drugs? What if our thoughts and moods are influenced by what we eat?

The increased prevalence of depression in Western populations has run parallel to fundamental alterations to the food supply. Food is not just an energy source; it is information. It contains instructions for our DNA and can turn our genes on or off, alter hormones such as cortisol, insulin and serotonin, and sex hormones, and change the composition of our gut microbiome. The influence of food on the health and wellness of our mind is now in the spotlight — and it's about time.

Sometimes effects of food (or lack of nutrients) can be extreme, but altered very easily. Patients have presented with manifestations of mood disorders — as serious as hallucinations and suicidal tendencies — and then symptoms are identified as a result of a vitamin B12 deficiency. For example, a sixteen-year-old male who presented with irritability, regressive behaviour, apathy, hallucinations and suicidal thoughts was found to be deficient in B12. The symptoms of mixed mood disorder remediated immediately after supplementation,[46] demonstrating just how meaningful the relationship between nutritional status and a healthy mind is.

We know that nutritional status impacts the gut microbiome and there is a link between our gut, inflammation and mental health. Recent research from the journal *Nature Microbiology* showed a strong relationship between microbiome health and mental health,[47] and inflammation and an unwell mind are intimately related.[48] We should not be merely concerned with warding off mental illness; rather, we need to be diligent in nourishing our mind with the right foods to improve our emotional wellbeing. If we are not eating foods that are rich in nutrients most of the time, our mind cannot produce the chemicals required to maintain a healthy mood.

Food is medicine for our mind.

Back to basics

I feel we have made a mess of the current nutritional landscape. Once we were hunter–gatherers, eating seasonally and locally from the land.[49] As mentioned, the Agricultural Revolution, followed by the Industrial Revolution, arose with far-reaching changes to the food supply. Rapidly growing world trade increased the amount and type of food available, and this continued at an even greater pace after World War II.

Fast forward to modern day. Our highly processed food supply is riddled with chemicals and pesticides from industrialized agriculture. And, industrialized agriculture focuses on a few monocrops, which in turn degrades our soil, leading to nutrient depletion (but that's a topic for another book). We then add salt, sugar and chemical additives to our food, in the name of taste and convenience. Let's delve a little further into what has changed and why it may impact the health and wellbeing of our mind.

Loren Cordain and colleagues have highlighted that before the development of agriculture, we consumed foods straight from the ground, including hundreds of different types of fruits and vegetables. This dropped substantially after the introduction of grains. Cereals and bread then became a staple, displacing fruits and vegetables as a primary source of energy. Additionally, meat intake from grass-fed and wild sources was replaced by grain-fed varieties of livestock. Animals do not thrive on grains; rather, they get fat and have a range of health problems as a result. Antibiotics are the treatment of choice for the sick animals and this is now a public health concern, because there is speculation that eating animals treated with antibiotics impacts human health. While evidence is scant (for now) that the current increase in resistant strains of bacteria is a direct result of agricultural antibiotic use, concern is still warranted.[50]

Convenience versus wellbeing

As technology has advanced, so has the crusade to provide consumers what we seemingly desire most: convenience. Starting with the proliferation of canned and frozen foods in the 1920s, we now have what can only be described as 'fake food' wrapped in cardboard and plastic (as if the world doesn't have enough challenges!). Yes, I get it: time is valuable, and who has time to spend in the kitchen? People who value their emotional and mental wellbeing, and their physical health and wellbeing — and that of their family. That's who!

I have little spare time, and would much prefer convenience over 40–60 minutes of preparing and cooking food each day. However, I am aware of how my mind functions on a diet of processed foods, and conversely on a diet of nutritious, whole foods. Consequently, I have chosen to prioritize and invest the time. I highly recommend you too invest your time in nourishing your body and brain.

The manipulation

Processed foods are designed to make us crave more. In fact, food manufacturers count on it and strive to provide processed foods that contain more fat, salt and sugar; our appetite gravitates towards these nutrients for survival. We then eat more, as processed foods trigger reward centres in our brain, which compromise our health.[51]

I was researching salt taste sensitivity and the intake of high sodium foods early in my research career. During my investigation I discovered that food manufacturers spend time assessing the saltiness (for example) required to ensure preference and intake by consumers. They do the testing in a sensory booth in a laboratory setting. The outcome of my study suggests that people will be satisfied with lower concentrations of sodium contained in a processed food when they are eating a meal in a social situation, rather than when in a laboratory setting.[52] This makes sense, doesn't it? When we eat foods as part of a meal the flavours work together in a synergistic manner, so realistically food manufacturers could reduce the sodium concentration significantly without any impact to the acceptance of the food. Unfortunately, we also adapt to sodium concentration in food. So, as food manufacturers add more sodium to satisfy perceived taste preferences, consumers then want more sodium in their processed foods.

Processed foods may taste good (remember, much work has gone into making them taste amazing to hook us in), and may save us time. However, they do not contribute to health and wellbeing. We need to be responsible and take control for the health of our mind and not hand over our control to food manufacturers.

Who wants to walk through life in a meat suit filled with rubbish posing as food?

We need to change our ways

Several studies coming out from the Deakin University, Mood and Food Centre,[53] have strongly suggested that diets with a high intake of processed food are associated with increased anxiety and depression,[54] while dietary patterns consisting of high intake of vegetables, fruits, nuts, seeds and fatty fish reduce the risk of mood disorders.[55] This is in line with a Mediterranean-style dietary pattern, which has recently been shown to improve mental health when supplemented with fish oil.[56]

Not only do foods change the health of our brain, they alter its very structures. New research has found that high levels of Propionic Acid (PPA) — which increases the shelf life of packaged foods, and inhibits mould in processed cheese and bread — negatively impacts the development of neurons in unborn babies.[57] Associate Professor Felice Jacka, director of the Mood and Food Centre, has stated that a diet containing large amounts of highly processed foods leads to a smaller hippocampus, an area of our brain important for mood regulation.[58] What we eat changes the structure of our brain.

Diet quality and depression

The SMILES trial,[59] which involved participants suffering major depression, looks at the effects of improved diet quality on mental wellbeing. This first randomised control trial has reported that depression is alleviated in those with a better quality diet.

Sixty-seven participants were enrolled in the study, over twelve weeks. The predominant aim of the study was to increase diet quality by encouraging the intake of twelve key food groups (recommended servings in brackets):

- whole grains (five–eight servings per day)

- vegetables (six per day)

- fruit (three per day)

- legumes (three–four per week)

- low-fat and unsweetened dairy foods (two–three per day)

- raw and unsalted nuts (one per day)

- fish (at least two per week)

- lean red meats (three–four per week)

- chicken (two–three per week)

- eggs (up to six per week)

- virgin olive oil (three tablespoons per day).

Extra foods, such as sweets, refined cereals, fried food, fast food, processed meats and sugary drinks (no more than three per week), were significantly reduced. Red or white wine consumption beyond two standard drinks per day and all other alcohol (e.g. spirits, beer) were included within an extras food group. Study participants were advised to consume red wine if drinking alcohol, and only drink with meals.

The results are impressive to date, with significant reductions in symptoms, suggesting that improvements to diet quality will enhance the health of our mind and ease depressive symptoms. In addition to this randomized control trial, there are observational studies supporting the notion that the quality of our food impacts the health and wellbeing of our mind.[60]

Quality of food doesn't only relate to nutritional density, but also variety.

Variety is key

Of course we know that fruit and vegetable intake is related to better brain health,[61] but consuming a *variety* of these foods is also important. For a healthy mind, high intake and a large array of vegetables is best.

Dr Terry Wahls, author of *The Wahls Protocol*,[62] was a typical physician who prescribed drugs for most ailments, until she wound up with Multiple Sclerosis. The disease took hold and Wahls quickly became confined to a tilt-recline wheelchair. She took the usual medications that she prescribed to her patients, but she only got worse. Then, she had an epiphany: conventional medicine was failing her. After researching the foods that would nourish her brain, she embraced a paleo-style diet with grass-fed meat, wild fish and a range of vegetables. In fact, she now includes 9 cups of green and leafy vegetables, sulphur-rich vegetables and brightly coloured vegetables every day. This enabled Wahls to regain control of her health. Within months she had ditched the wheelchair, was out bike riding daily, as well as tossing all of her disease-modifying drugs. On recalling her research, Wahls states:

I learned that when we eat more sugar, processed foods and white flour-based foods, we are more likely to have a mix of bacteria associated with worse health. Whereas a diet with nine serves of vegetables a day is more likely to have a mix of microbes associated with better health outcomes.

I then created a diet for my brain, based on research, to provide what my brain needed and looked at implementing stress-reducing activities. The idea was to create a healthy environment for my brain and optimize the environmental factors that might work to help me achieve my greatest health.[63]

But how do we create a healthy environment — in terms of nutrition — for our brain when diet wars are raging all around us, and nutrition is so confusing?

It's not hard

Good nutrition shouldn't come down to whether you embrace a paleo, keto, vegan, gluten-free or any new frilly, fanciful approach to nutrition. Optimal nutrition is about a variety of high-quality, nutrient-dense unprocessed foods that are grown naturally and sustainably. It is simple, we need to go back to basics.

Eating healthy, organic food can be expensive. And cooking from scratch is costly for the time poor. I recommend that you buy organic produce where possible, due to the confirmed detrimental effects of glyphosate on health (see below), but why not consider growing your own food if you have the capacity? It's not only healthy and inexpensive — it's incredibly satisfying. Eating a 'mind changing' diet involves consuming food either grown in the ground, fed by the ground, or living in the sea.

~

Glyphosate — stop consuming it!

Glyphosate (Roundup, the weed killer) began its spree in 1974 and is now the most heavily used pesticide globally. We even use it in our home gardens! Many studies suggest links between glyphosate and cancer,[64] kidney disease,[65] infertility[66] and more. As a herbicide, glyphosate disrupts EPSPS, a specific plant enzyme in the shikimate pathway, resulting in protein shortage and eventual death. Animals do not have the shikimate pathway, but plants and bacteria do. It has been suggested that glyphosate may be damaging our intestinal microbiome due to its pernicious effects on bacteria, although to date there are conflicting results.

Regardless, we don't want to be eating foods covered in glyphosate. It is so prevalent that a study found between 0.210 and 0.432 nanograms per millilitre in breast milk.[67] Drinking water is allowed to have no more than 0.100 nanograms of glyphosate. It needs to be noted that the study conducted on breast milk was not peer reviewed and therefore results should be approached with caution.

On another note, it appears the use of glyphosate is affecting the gut bacteria in bees, leaving them at risk of malnourishment and infection. We need pollinators such as bees to help plants survive, and we need plants for nutrients.

The six-ingredient rule

This is simple: do not eat anything with more than six ingredients. And stay away from ingredients you can't pronounce.

Take the humble loaf of bread. I don't eat much bread. Not because I am gluten intolerant, but rather I want to reduce any diet-induced inflammation. When I do eat bread I eat a sourdough containing:

- organic wholemeal spelt flour
- filtered water
- olive oil
- sea salt
- sourdough culture (gut-loving probiotics).

Five ingredients. This bread does cost a little more than other commercial breads, but it's a cost I am willing to invest. Also it's dead easy to make! You can find plenty of sourdough recipes on the net: then you are in control of what goes into your bread, and into your body.

~

Usual bread ingredients

Wheat Flour, Water, Yeast, Vinegar, Iodized Salt, Canola Oil, Soy Flour, Vegetable Emulsifier (471, 481, 472e), Mineral Salt (Calcium Carbonate), Vitamins (Thiamin, Folic Acid)

If you feel the need for 'real' bread, I recommend sourdough due to its long fermentation process. This may reduce the toxicity of gluten,[68] for those who are sensitive, and may also increase magnesium and phosphorus.[69] A big issue with some breads is that they contain emulsifiers, and emerging evidence suggests that these plunder and destroy our healthy gut microbiome, which in turn impact mood and mind.[70]

Read labels

The next rule: always read food labels. We can easily be misled by labels like 'low sugar', 'healthy' or 'low GMO', especially with those standout fonts and multiple stars. A recent Australian study reported that seven out of ten packaged foods contain sugars that are not clearly identified on the label.[71] Even nutrition experts can get confused!

Especially look out for labels with the following:

- dextrose
- fructose
- galactose
- glucose (and plenty of other oses)
- corn syrup
- high fructose syrup

- barley malt extract

- rice malt syrup

- agave

- coconut sugar

- palm sugar

- any fruit concentrate such as grape fruit concentrate or treacle.

These are all sugars. Check out what is listed in the first three ingredients of the food you are considering buying. If it is any of the above listed, then the food is very high in added sugar and should be avoided. We will discuss the impact of sugar on our health shortly.

Sugar isn't the only food to check for when examining labels. Don't be fooled by 'all natural' — many foods described as all natural have preservatives, or high fructose corn syrup added (high fructose corn syrup is not a problem in Australia but is used frequently in the United States and other countries that have abundant access to maize). 'All natural' is not defined by the Food and Drug Administration,[72] and so there is flexibility for manufacturers to add non-natural products.

Foods labelled as 'low fat' or 'fat free' don't mean healthy. A food labelled '97 percent fat free' is still 3 percent fat. (And we will discuss that vegetable oil is not favourable in the next section.) For a food to claim that it is fat free, it must have less than 0.15 percent fat.

Fat free is often in large text on the front of confectionary labels to grab our attention away from the reality that we are about to ingest large concentrations of sugar instead.

Foods labelled 'no added sugar' can also be misleading, because the food may contain natural sugars such as fructose. For example, pear juice concentrate is often added as a sweetener but has just as many kilojoules as refined sugar.

Ignore claims of 'no cholesterol' as cholesterol from foods is not important. There is no relationship between cholesterol in food, blood cholesterol levels and heart disease — this was debunked a while ago.[73] The body produces cholesterol and can clear out excess cholesterol, when functioning properly. Rather sugar[74] and trans fats[75] play a role in raising blood cholesterol.

How many of us are enticed with the words 'baked, not fried'? This does not mean low in fat, but somehow it just sounds healthier, right? The baked potato chips may have less fat, but if it has more than 25 percent fat it is not considered low. Also, baked chips are also one of the highest sources of acrylamide, which is a carcinogenic chemical that can form when high-carbohydrate foods — such as potatoes — are heated to high temperatures. The FDA found that baked potato chips contain about three times more acrylamide than traditional fried chips.[76]

It's really important to take ownership of what you put into your body: it is empowering and plays a role in taking control of the health of your mind. One way to achieve this is by reading labels to ensure that any manufactured foods we choose to consume are not harming our body and mind.

Additives

Natural food additives and chemicals can provoke reactions in some people. Sulphates, glutamate, salicylate and amines can produce severe reactions and have vastly different effects on different people. If we are to eliminate foods containing natural chemicals, a total revamp of the diet is required. For most, this is a deterrent unless symptoms are significantly problematic. The potential effects of naturally occurring chemicals on the mind should be considered on an individual basis, with avoidance of a strict exclusion approach, which may result in nutrient depletion in some. So, please consult a dietician or nutritionist before attempting any strict exclusion diet.

A review conducted in 2015 by Isabel Skypala and colleagues[77] lists foods high in added and naturally occurring chemicals that potentially cause sensitivities in some people, with advice that removal of a few of these high-risk foods is a wiser approach than a severe exclusion diet; a table reproduced from this study with foods listed is below. If you feel that food sensitivities are influencing the health of your mind, please seek advice from an expert in food sensitivities. The gold standard for identifying problem foods is an elimination diet for a couple of weeks, and then gradual reintroduction of foods to identify the culprit.

Amine, glutamate, salicylate and sulphate table

Food	Amine	Glutamate	Salicylate	Sulphate
Cheese	✓	✓		
Wine	✓		✓	✓
Soy	✓	✓		
Tea		✓	✓	
Food	Amine	Glutamate	Salicylate	Sulphate
Tomatoes	✓	✓	✓	
Herbs and spices			✓	
Strawberries and pineapple	✓		✓	
Spinach	✓	✓		
Worcestershire sauce		✓	✓	
Dried fruit			✓	✓

The topic of food additives and colouring is controversial to say the least. Several food regulatory departments, as well as the Dieticians Association of Australia (DAA) claim that food additives are safe for most people.[78]

I argue that there is evidence that artificial sweeteners and emulsifiers are linked to inflammation and alterations to our gut microbiome,[79] and a recent study conducted by Lucia Hrncirova and colleagues has shown that our microbiome is highly susceptible to sodium benzoate (commonly used to conserve margarine, pickles, salad dressings, juices and carbonated drinks), sodium nitrite (used to conserve processed fish and meat products such as bacon) and potassium sorbate (used in cheese, cakes, ice-cream, soft drinks and syrups).[80] The authors concede that modified gut microbiome caused by food additives may result in the increased prevalence of autoimmune disease. I would raise the question: could alterations in gut microbiome resulting from additives in processed foods increase prevalence of illness of the mind? Mary Holder and colleagues have recently published an article showing that emulsifiers are linked with anxiety-related behaviours in mice,[81] and human studies will, I hope, follow.

Optimal diet for mental wellness?

As I noted, nutrition is confusing and I don't subscribe to a one-size-fits-all approach. We all have different nutritional requirements at different times in our life and the most important factor is nutrient density, not calories. However, you can use dietary strategies that are grounded in strong research to facilitate a well mind.

The scope of this book does not extend to individual diet plans. Rather it takes a pragmatic approach and provides advice for sourcing food to nourish the mind. If you suspect you suffer food sensitivities, seek a screening with your health practitioner or book in with a nutritionist or dietician for individualized advice.

If you're becoming too restrictive and obsessive with food choices, and your dietary patterns are causing feelings of anxiety, it's time to take stock. Get some advice from a nutritionist or dietician.

While I support the aim to eat an unprocessed and as-natural-as-possible diet, this should not be at the expense of peace of mind, or important nutrients. An obsession with eating the right kind of foods can be an eating disorder in disguise. Eating exclusively keto, paleo or raw food can result in missing out on essential nutrients, and also an element of joy associated with sharing food with others.

I want you to approach food as a gift from nature and nourishment for your body and mind. What we feed ourselves reflects self-care; a fundamental component of a well mind.

CHAPTER 7:

Inflammation

'We are living in a world today where lemonade
is made from artificial flavours and furniture
polish is made from real lemons.'

Alfred E Newman

Henry Cotton was an American psychiatrist who moved up the ranks
to be medical doctor and superintendent of the Trenton Psychiatric
hospital in 1907. What set Cotton apart from his colleagues was
that he was convinced that insanity originated from untreated
infections in the body.[82]

What followed was macabre to say the least. Cotton began by
removing infected teeth from his patients. If that didn't work, he
went to work on other infected body parts. Tonsils, ovaries, colons,
you name it — if it was infected, out it came.

Cotton reported an 85 percent remission rate in his patients (they may not have had all of their teeth or organs intact but they weren't crazy or depressed anymore). His success rate drew interest from his colleagues but after his death in 1933, interest in the inflammation theory for mental illness waned. The mortality rates from Cotton's bizarre approach sat at a devastating 45 percent and his hypothesis was discredited. Fast forward to the 21st century and a growing body of research highlights that there might be some truth to Cotton's belief that infection (followed by inflammation) is the precursor to an unwell mind.

In 2014 a review published by Turhan Canli, professor of integrative neuroscience, argued that major depression is birthed in bacterial, viral or parasitic infection.[83] What stands out about his paper is that, similar to Cotton, Canli suggests reframing major depression as an infectious disease as opposed to an emotional disorder (with no mention of removing infected teeth or organs, thankfully).

Even when we have the flu our immune response goes into overdrive. Proteins and proinflammatory mediators generate an immune response that promotes symptoms that make us want to curl up and sleep all day. And importantly, the blood–brain barrier is not as impenetrable as once believed,[84] so inflammatory proteins can enter the brain and create an inflammatory cascade. That's right: you may have an inflammatory response in your body and that response will reach your brain and cause inflammation in your mind.

In her book *Brain on Fire: My Month of Madness*[85] journalist Susannah Cahalan recounts her experience after an inflammatory reaction prompted by a rare neurological disorder left her with paranoid delusions and hallucinations. Fortunately, after her team of physicians failed to diagnose her during psychosis, a new neurologist joined the team and recognized the symptoms. He identified a recently discovered autoimmune disorder in which the body attacks the brain, a disease now thought to be tied to both schizophrenia and autism, and perhaps was responsible for apparent 'demonic possessions' recorded throughout history.

We are often told that mental illness is a chemical imbalance in our brain with no mention of inflammation. But no human trial has ever indicated any imbalance of serotonin (or other chemical).[86] Rather, the amygdala and the prefrontal cortex can be affected by inflammation, and therefore emotions may become dysregulated.[87] And the last thing we need is our emotional health being bulldozed, because emotional health affects everything from our relationships to even our ability to get out of bed in the morning. We have to calm the immune system down by reducing inflammation, but how do we do that? Nature has gifted us powerful anti-inflammatory compounds in foods; however, because we are dumb humans, we have also created several inflammatory foods that only cause us harm in body and mind.

The bad stuff

Listed below are foods that have a terrible effect on our mind, and they are scattered throughout the Western food supply.

Seed oils

We can identify processed foods by the dietary fat quality. The presence of seed oils (which were a lovely 'gift' from the Industrial Revolution) is verification that the food is processed, and not natural. Anything containing canola, soybean, sunflower oil or any other industrial seed oil will not nourish and heal your body or brain. These oils contain polyunsaturated fatty acids that oxidise easily and are unstable. This can then lead to the production of lipid peroxides and trans fats, which are highly inflammatory.[88]

~

Avoid PolyUnsaturated Fatty Acids (PUFA)

All fats have a temperature at which they oxidise (become unstable, rancid and toxic). The temperature that this occurs when using PUFAs is very low. Unstable fats are prone to oxidation, which leads to free radicals, which are responsible for damaging your cells and accelerating aging. Oxidised fatty acids are highly inflammatory. In one study, researchers oxidised some soybean oil by heating it up several times and then fed it to rats. The oxidised soybean oil caused inflammation and promoted hypertension.[89]

Seed oils have a high ratio of omega-6 fatty acids, as do grains. The use of such oils has contributed to a decrease in our dietary intake of omega-3 fatty acids (anti-inflammatory), and has increased omega-6 fatty acids (pro-inflammatory). Having evolved on a ratio of 1:1 for these fatty acids, now we consume far greater amounts of omega-6 than omega-3s. Increased omega-6 fatty acids are linked with a number of chronic diseases, and a significant increase in inflammation.[90] So, the modern diet, with high grain intake, reliance on vegetable and seed oils, and the switch from grass-fed animals to grain-fed sources of meat, has led us to a pro-inflammatory disaster zone. And to reiterate, diet-induced inflammation is intimately related to the health of our mind.

Trans Fats

Seed oils are sometimes hydrogenated — think of a nice yellow cake of margarine. When this occurs we end up with a food containing trans fatty acids. If you see 'partially hydrogenated' on the food label, run for dear life.

Trans fats are detrimental to a healthy mind. A study conducted in Spain reported that those who had higher levels of trans fats in their blood have a 48 percent increased risk of depression.[91] Additionally, another study highlighted that a diet high in trans fats is linked to anger and irritability.[92] And a recent study found that these fatty acids are strongly related to anxiety and depression in older adults.[93]

Trans fatty acids are kryptonite for a well mind, and once you start looking you'll find them in many supermarket items. Margarine, popcorn (you know the disgusting butter-flavoured microwave stuff), doughnuts, pastries, cinnamon scrolls, French fries, hash browns, pies, pasties, sausage rolls, quiches, bagels — all have trans fats in them.

Sugar

You knew this was coming, didn't you? Sugar is toxic for the mind, just as it is for the body.

I recall my daughter telling me once that her husband could pick when she had binged on chocolate because her moods were all over the place. And I experience the same (unrelated to bipolar, I can assure you). A study by Isabelle Aeberli and colleagues involving 29 healthy adults, highlights that consuming sugary drink increases inflammatory markers,[94] and inflammation impacts our mood.[95] So, it's not just the rollercoaster effect of blood sugar levels on mood we need to be wary of.

When we eat sugary foods, the reward centres in the brain are activated and we get a massive hit of dopamine (the neurotransmitter linked to pleasure and reward also plays a role in addiction). Eating sugar makes us feel so good and it acts as a powerful, incredibly addictive and harmful drug.

While it is true that we used to obtain sugar from seasonal fruit picking in hunter–gatherer times, the sweet, refined white stuff in virtually all processed foods now was not part of our diet. Not until the Middle Ages did the processed version become popular in Europe, and even then it was considered too expensive for everyday consumption. So, for the majority of our existence as a species, processed sugar simply didn't rate. We have a sweet tooth to encourage us to crave the nutrient-dense, energy-giving fruits that were available in short supply, in season, in the ancestral food supply. But now sugar is plentiful and we still crave it. Westerners eat more than a kilo of sugar a week compared to practically none 150 years ago.[96]

As I have mentioned, refined sugar is highly inflammatory.[97] When our blood sugar rises, the body fires out greater numbers of pro-inflammatory molecules called cytokines, and if we are eating it daily we will be in a constant state of low-grade or chronic inflammation.

And, another big deal is that sugar intake is associated with poor gut health. Eating processed, sugar-laden foods negatively impacts the community of our gut flora.[98] The bad bacteria in our gut love sugar, and it has been well documented that a high intake of sugar alters the balance of good versus bad bacteria. When the bad guys in our gut overrun the good, all kinds of nasty effects take place.

One is that the gut mucosa (the lining of our gut that plays a vital role as a barrier for our intestine) deviates from normal.[99] When the gut mucosa is altered, increased gut permeability may arise — and the dreaded leaky gut syndrome follows. Leaky gut is when the tight mesh in the gut membrane loosens after exposure to unhealthy foods, also inflammatory foods such as gluten. Consequently, partially digested food, toxins and bacteria can then penetrate the tissues beneath the membrane and enter the blood circulation. These toxic substances entering the blood can cause an autoimmune response and create an inflammatory fire that not only affects our body, but also our mind.[100] More on a leaky gut later.

Gluten

Dietary patterns that promote inflammation are high in refined sugar, starches and trans fats. We may as well just refer to it as a Western diet (high in processed meats, baked goods and refined grains).[101] I mentioned earlier that I personally avoid gluten (which is difficult to do these days), and I am not gluten intolerant. The reason I do this is because many studies have demonstrated that it is highly inflammatory.[102]

Some reports claim that gluten can promote inflammation in the brain, but I have not encountered any worthwhile research that confirms this — yet. However, anecdotal evidence does suggest that when gluten is eliminated, symptoms such as brain fog, depression and anxiety do alleviate.

Dr David Perlmutter, mentioned earlier, also wrote *Grain Brain*, in which he documented a case study of a nine-year-old girl brought by her parents to see him, primarily because she had poor memory.

Perlmutter was told that the girl had difficulty thinking and focusing, and was struggling at school. Her parents indicated that she couldn't keep thoughts together, and that as a result she was often frustrated.

After some testing Perlmutter reported that the girl's neurological examinations were entirely normal, and the typical blood tests were unrevealing. So, they were left with a mystery. Considering that the girl apparently had segments of time where she was functioning well, Perlmutter concluded that her brain was intact but that something sinister was affecting her mind intermittently. Diet was the first factor investigated, because it can change on a day-to-day basis.

Because gluten sensitivity is common, Perlmutter tested to see if the girl was gluten sensitive, and she was. She was put on a gluten-free diet (which is really challenging if you tend to drool walking past your local bakery), and all wheat, barley and rye was eliminated. Within a couple of weeks the parents reported positive results. She could suddenly focus far easier on her school work and told her parents that she noticed she was thinking much more clearly. She stayed gluten-free over the next several months and continued to notice further improvements in her school work.[103]

As far back as 1996, Dr Marios Hadjivassiliou, a world authority on gluten sensitivity, reported that 'gluten sensitivity can primarily be considered a neurological disease'.[104] It seems that antibodies that a person possesses when sensitive to gluten can be directly and uniquely toxic to the brain.

A review published in *The New England Journal of Medicine* listed 55 diseases resulting from gluten intake, including anxiety, depression and schizophrenia.[105]

~

How to test for gluten sensitivity

Coeliac disease — an allergy to gluten — is different to gluten sensitivity. Changes in the blood can be seen when a person is allergic to gluten; however, for gluten sensitivity, no test exists. Before gluten sensitivity can be diagnosed, coeliac disease must be ruled out, so a panel of blood tests will be conducted to look for the antibodies that indicate the condition. There is some evidence that two of the tests on the coeliac disease panel — the AGA-IgA and the AGG-IgG — could indicate non-coeliac gluten sensitivity as well. However, because no test can yield conclusive results, the best method to determine sensitivity is to remove gluten from the diet and observe if symptoms abate.

This is a controversial area, and as mentioned I refrain where possible from consuming gluten. I have observed an improvement in my mood when experimenting with exclusion of dietary gluten, but of course this is my experience and may not apply to all.

The good stuff

Listed below are foods that are important to include in your daily diet for a well mind, and they are anti-inflammatory.

Omega-3 Fatty Acids

It has been fifteen years since it was first suggested that increasing omega-3 fatty acid intake has a beneficial effect on the mind. Since then, many studies have found omega-3 to be helpful in alleviating depression and anxiety.[106] But how is this possible? Omega-3s easily travel through the brain cell membrane and interact with mood-related chemicals inside the brain. They also have anti-inflammatory actions that may help prevent and alleviate mood disorders.

In saying that, one review states that results are inconclusive, and that the benefits of omega-3 (think high intake of fish) may also be impacted by overall diet quality and lifestyle factors.[107] This makes sense, because good health is comprised of several lifestyle factors. The traditional Mediterranean diet has a high fish intake,[108] and much evidence suggests that this dietary pattern reduces risk of depression. In fact, a recent systematic review and meta-analysis published in the journal *Molecular Psychiatry* concludes that adhering to a Mediterranean-style diet and avoiding a pro-inflammatory diet offers protection against depression.[109]

Importantly, omega-3 fatty acids are anti-inflammatory, and that is our goal for a well mind — to reduce inflammation.

~

Omega-3s in your diet

Foods that provide omega-3 fatty acids:

- Fatty fish (salmon, mackerel, sardines, oysters, trout)

- Nuts and seeds (walnuts, pecans, hazelnuts, flaxseed, chia seeds, hemp seeds)

- Supplements (krill oil, fish oil, cod liver oil, algae oil).

Virgin olive oil

Extra-virgin olive oil is made from pure, cold-pressed olives, and is the highest quality oil. Virgin olive oil is also unrefined and of high quality, whereas plain old olive oil is a blend that includes a mixture of cold-pressed and refined processed oils. Always choose extra-virgin or virgin olive oil for purity and so you obtain a high concentration of phenolic compounds.

Extra-virgin, or virgin olive oil has plenty of anti-inflammatory properties. In my PhD thesis I covered the anti-inflammatory actions of oleocanthal, a phenolic compound in virgin olive oil. Among the various and wide-reaching health benefits of virgin olive oil consumption, it seems it is also beneficial for a healthy mind.

The SMILES study mentioned earlier (see page 86), gave participants three tablespoons of virgin olive oil a day and saw reductions in symptoms of depression. Because the oil has many phenolic compounds, most of which are anti-inflammatory (especially oleocanthal),[110] virgin olive oil should be included in a healthy-mind diet. A good quality virgin olive oil is packed to the brim with powerful antioxidants and anti-inflammatory agents, so literally pour it over all of your food!

~

Virgin olive oil on everything

Dr Steven Gundry, a former cardiac surgeon and author, suggests consuming three tablespoons of virgin olive oil per day. Pour it on vegetables and salads, or just consume straight up. A good virgin olive oil will burn your throat a little, and this is due to the beneficial compound oleocanthal.

Saturated fat

Nature has provided us with many foods with potent anti-inflammatory properties. And we have also been led to believe that some foods are healthy when they are in fact unhealthy, and vice versa. So, how do we know what's true? I'm not going to include saturated fat as a 'good fat'. But let's un-demonize it.

Saturated fat has had a shockingly bad rap for promoting risk of cardiovascular disease. But, it seems this is not correct. Many studies are now showing that saturated fat (alone, not mixed with nice sugary burger buns at Maccas) is not evil after all.[111] Saturated fats from pasture-raised meats contain vitamins A, D and K2, and any reported benefits of replacing saturated fat with carbohydrate have been well challenged.[112] I had always been taught that we should reduce saturated fat intake and increase carbohydrate intake for good health, and so that is what I did. During this time my mind was really unwell.

It all started back in the 1970s when the Seven Countries Study[113] was published, purporting that saturated fat is linked to heart disease. The study didn't take into consideration sugar intake, or other factors such as smoking and exercise; therefore, it was flawed from the outset. And there are suggestions that countries with high saturated fat intake and no incidence of heart disease were excluded from the analysis. Our dietary guidelines were formulated on this foundation, with recommendations for low fat, high carbohydrate intake following. We are only now starting to raise questions regarding this approach, which is clearly not working.

Many studies suggesting that saturated fat is unhealthy are conducted in the presence of refined carbohydrate — and we now know that in combination, sugar and fat is like a dysfunctional marriage. We are seeing more and more evidence that refined carbohydrates (refined is key here), are linked to greater adverse health effects.[114] This isn't to say you should go out and have bacon and eggs daily — bacon is a processed meat, and nitrates in processed meats are carcinogenic — however, saturated fats in *moderation* such as coconut oil, butter and pasteurized eggs are now considered healthy foods.

Berries

Anti-inflammatory fruits are gold. I love berries, especially blue ones. These awesome little nutrient balls contain polyphenol compounds that promote potent anti-inflammatory activity in humans. Anthocyanins create the distinctive colours of red, blue and purple and are the anti-inflammatory superhero of the berry, because they modulate inflammatory pathways,[115] and they are packed with antioxidants. When you eat blueberries and wind up with blue lips, it's the anthocyanins that are to blame. Strawberries are a really great addition as snacks or dessert and have been shown to have powerful anti-inflammatory actions.[116]

~

Eat your berries

Aim for 1 cup of fresh or frozen berries a day. If you can't access fresh organic berries, soak non-organic ones in apple cider vinegar (four parts water, one part apple cider vinegar) in a bowl for at least 30 minutes and then rinse. This will help get rid of any pesticides; berries are one of the dirty dozen foods carrying the highest concentration of pesticides.

Vegetables

'Eat all your veggies,' I was told repeatedly as a child, then I said it to my kids, I say it to my stepkids, and I also now say it back to my mum. And we all know that we say it because vegetables are good for us. But we haven't really grasped that the incredible health benefits extend to the mind. Recent studies have highlighted that fruit and vegetable intake are linked to greater mental wellbeing. [117]

Vegetables give us loads of crucial nutrients and fibre. Cruciferous vegetables such as cabbage, cauliflower, kale, radishes, bok choy, broccoli and Brussels sprouts contain important compounds known as isothiocyanates and indoles, which can prevent oxidative damage. These vegetables, as well as spinach and lettuce, also contain the vitamins A, B, C and K.

Cabbage, broccoli, cauliflower, onions, garlic, mushrooms and asparagus all contain sulphur; yup, the stuff that smells like rotten eggs. Dr Terry Wahls (see page 87) includes sulphur-rich vegetables in her protocol because sulphur is required for the synthesis of glutathione, one of the most powerful antioxidants we have.[118] High glutathione levels are associated with excellent mental health, and have been shown to alleviate many mind disorders such as bipolar, depression, anxiety and autism.[119]

Avocado

The avo has been worshipped as a good-mood food for a while now, and with good reason. The creamy goodness of an avocado contains tryptophan, which is a precursor to serotonin: our 'feel-good' chemical. An avocado also contains omega-3 fatty acids and important B vitamins, which are all really healthful for our brain, and they have anti-inflammatory properties.

The human brain is nearly 60 percent fat, so eating a fruit so full of monounsaturated fat like an avocado is incredibly nourishing.[120]

Turmeric

Turmeric is an ancient spice that has been used in Chinese and ayurvedic medicine for centuries. Curcuminoids in turmeric have anti-inflammatory properties inhibiting both the activity and the synthesis of pro-inflammatory cyclooxygenase-2 (COX2) and 5-lipoxygenase (5-LOX), as well as other enzymes linked to inflammation.[121] Adding turmeric to your diet also enhances the synthesis of omega-3 docosahexaenoic acid (DHA) from its precursor, α-linolenic acid (ALA), according to a study from the UCLA Brain Injury Research Centre.[122] Evidence also suggests that this 'super' spice can alleviate symptoms of depression.[123]

Because of its anti-inflammatory actions, turmeric should certainly be added to the 'mind changing' arsenal. However, a note before you believe that turmeric will leave you inflammation free; curcumin — the compound that gives turmeric its wondrous properties — isn't particularly bioavailable, meaning that after ingestion not much gets into the system and so can't be used by the body.

Regardless, there is evidence of its efficacy in humans when combined with other compounds to improve bioavailability. A recent study from the *Chinese Journal of Integrative Medicine* reported that curcumin was helpful in reducing anxiety in a sample of obese adults. The randomized double blind cross-over trial involved participants consuming curcumin as 500-mg C3 Complex® (standardized powder extract obtained from Alleppey finger turmeric containing a minimum 95 percent concentration of three curcuminoids: curcumin, bisdemethoxycurcumin and demethoxycurcumin) plus 5 mg bioperine® per serving to enhance absorption.[124] Participants took the supplement for four weeks, and those taking the bioavailable curcumin had significantly lower anxiety scores compared to placebo group.

And, of importance, a recent pilot study found that those who took a turmeric and black-pepper supplement experienced a 7 percent increase in gut microbiome diversity, with the researchers claiming that turmeric had a prebiotic effect by helping local bacteria and other microorganisms thrive.[125] Which leads us to the connection between gut health and our brain.

CHAPTER 8:

The Gut

'If there's one thing to know about the human body, it's this: the human body has a ringmaster. This ringmaster controls your digestion, your immunity, your brain, your weight, your health and even your happiness. This ringmaster is the gut.'

Nancy Mure

Karen recalled the first time she identified a connection between bloating and other gastrointestinal discomfort with her anxiety. It was the time she was asked to present at a conference her company was hosting. She always got nervous at the prospect of public speaking. Six weeks before her presentation she felt a familiar queasy feeling in her stomach, which made her even more anxious. Karen had experienced sensitivities to food previously, so she knew what was coming. To her dismay this time was no different; if anything, it was worse.

Everything Karen consumed resulted in constipation and horrendous pain, to the point that eventually she became too afraid to eat anything other than bland foods. This left her malnourished after a month, because her body was not obtaining enough nutrients from the only foods that she felt comfortable to eat.

Because this had been a pattern over the years her nutritional diversity was low. Therefore, Karen was depleting her gut bacteria, and so microbial diversity in her gut was also reduced. A key issue here is when the microbiome is depleted, the amygdala (again referring to the almond-shaped part of the brain that plays a role in anxiety; see page 71) becomes more highly branched and makes connections that it normally would not make, and so, Karen became more anxious. With that her fear of food became greater. She would do anything to reduce the gastrointestinal discomfort that she experienced and the fear of food then fuelled her anxiety, which only worsened her symptoms.

So, what do we do to avoid this dreadful scenario? Firstly Karen needed to incorporate some stress-mitigating practices such as meditation and breathwork (these will be covered soon). Acceptance that it would take some time to heal the gut is imperative in these situations. Karen had to get to a point where she believed she could heal her gut to reduce the debilitating anxiety that she endured. There is a feedback loop between mind and gut, which meant her mind also required attention.

Karen had to go back to basics in regards to diet, and she also needed to increase her microbial diversity. Because she had restricted her dietary intake to avoid the ongoing symptoms, Karen now needed to increase her nutrient intake to encourage healthy microbes.

She did this by adding different vegetables to her meals each day. For example, a big salad of spinach, cucumber, celery, carrots, snow peas, avocado and cranberries, dressed in lemon and virgin olive oil provided an array of vegetables that her gut microbiome would love, with healthy fats from the avocado and olive oil. Adding some fermented sauerkraut and a probiotic also helped get Karen's gut health back on track.

The gut microbiome

The inflammatory model of mental health has helped us appreciate the importance of the gut–brain connection. It's actually through the balance of the gut microbiome and the integrity of the gut lining that the brain receives signals from our external environment. If this goes awry, the brain is affected. The gut microbiome refers to the communities of microorganisms that live in your gut, and the balance of these communities is profoundly important for health and wellbeing.[126]

Our gut microbiome starts off as the colonization of flora from the mother's birth canal as we pass through it. Then colostrum given during the first feed, and later breast milk from the mother, adds more bacteria to the growing tribe of microbes. We then pick up microbes from contact with people and animals (and the odd pacifier dropped on the ground). Germs are generally good because they add to the diversity of flora in our gut throughout our lives. Exposure to different types of bacteria from birth develops gut immunity.

Toxins, exposure to antibiotics and processed foods create havoc for the poor little guys living in our gut. Because the microbiome has a fundamental role in absorbing nutrients, creating neurotransmitters and providing immunity, any dysregulation (or what we call dysbiosis — bad bacteria outweighing the good), will impact the connection between the gut and brain — referred to as the gut–brain axis.

Most research on gut health and depression involves rodents being injected with lipopolysaccharide (LPS), an endotoxin that is supposed to stay in the gut. Endotoxins make up the outer membrane of the cell wall in a gram-negative bacteria. Gram-negative bacteria include most of the bacteria found in the gastrointestinal tract, which cause infection and disease. If the gut lining is compromised in any way, LPS is often detected in the blood circulation, indicating that inflammation is present and causing an immune response. And in many cases when LPS and inflammation are present, illness of the mind follows.[127]

To digress briefly, I would like you to consider this. If we took a different approach and focused on measuring systemic inflammation first, rather than fixating on symptoms of mental illness, we could possibly uncover that we feel unwell in our mind because we are inflamed. Just a thought.

When we have discomfort in our gut, it can create discomfort in our mind. Therefore, the importance of the gut microbiome in mental wellness cannot be overstated.

There are more organisms in our gut than the number of people roaming the planet, and more than half of the human body is not human, rather microbial. We used to believe that everything was coded in our DNA. Back when the human genome project started we thought that the human genome would have around 250,000 functional genes to cover the complex range of processes that the human body is capable of. It turns out we may have fewer than 20,000 functional genes.[128] This is amazing when you compare a human to an insect, for example. We have so little genetic material, and we are about half as sophisticated as an earthworm, when looking at functional genes. In fact, the microbial genes that live in us account for most of our biological and metabolic activity. So much of our function is dictated by our microbiome, so we must take care of it.

A recent review I co-authored with colleagues from Swinburne University[129] highlights that stress influences the composition of gut microbiota. We discuss a study showing that emotional and environmental stressors such as maternal separation, crowding and heat can negatively impact the composition of gut microbiota in rodent studies.[130] In the study mice that were germ free (had no microbiome) had a more intense reaction to the stressors. What was interesting is that the stress response was decreased after oral administration of *bifidobacterium infantis* (a probiotic). This provides strong evidence that the microbiome has an important influence on the stress response.

A second brain

Just like the brain, the gut has its own nervous system, called the enteric nervous system (ENS). In fact, the gut contains more neurotransmitters than the brain! It is so complex and important that scientists are now calling it our 'second brain'. The ENS is made up of millions of neurons, with an entire ecosystem of bacteria communicating through, and with, the ENS. Crazy, right? Although our second brain doesn't reason, create or help us solve a mathematical equation, it does affect our mood state. And it is controlled by our gut microbiome.

~

Take care of your ENS

To take care of our second brain we need to nourish the gut microbiome with good quality and fermented foods, keep stress levels down, get quality carbohydrates from vegetables, and remove sugar and processed foods from the diet. Your diet is the most important factor to influence the gut microbiome, which is in control when it comes to the ENS and mood states.

The ENS receives signals from both sympathetic and parasympathetic nervous systems. The sympathetic nervous system is responsible for the fight-or-flight response. If, for example, you are swimming in the ocean and someone yells, 'Shark!' your heart rate will increase so that blood pumps to your muscles; your adrenal glands will be stimulated to produce adrenaline, which will ensure your liver releases glucose to fuel a quick escape; digestion will be inhibited; and the bronchioles in the lungs will dilate so you can take in more air to run (or in this case, swim). On the other hand, the parasympathetic nervous system will kick in when you reach the shore and realise that it was a false alarm. Your heart rate will slow; digestion will increase; and breathing will return to normal.

Of importance to the health of our mind is that the ENS should be receiving, and giving, signals from both the sympathetic and parasympathetic evenly — symmetrical signals keep you feeling even and balanced (something I struggled with for a long time). When one dominates, the sympathetic for example, you can be constantly stuck in fight-or-flight mode, and the chronic stress takes a toll and may manifest in the form of depression, anxiety, mania, or similar.

Another interesting element is that the ENS may trigger huge mood shifts experienced by people suffering with irritable bowel syndrome (IBS), or other ailments such as constipation, diarrhoea, bloating and pain. Who hasn't had at least one of those? Although it was believed for decades that anxiety and depression contribute to gastrointestinal issues, it seems it may be the other way around.

We are beginning to understand that inflammation and irritation in the gut signals to the central nervous system (CNS), which promotes mood imbalance, anxiety and depression.[131]

Leaky gut

Imagine a huge sheet of material — around 4000 square feet of surface area — forming a tight barrier that controls what enters and leaves your bloodstream: this is the gut lining. Certain foods, and also stress, alter the permeability of this lining so that larger molecules and endotoxins such as LPS can enter the circulation.[132]

Our immune response attacks quickly when foreign bodies are detected, which is helpful for survival. But, when the immune system garners all its weapons and attacks, fatalities occur in healthy cells as well. Because this goes on for a while it leads to low-grade inflammation, then an unwell mind, and an unwell mind can contribute to a leaky gut. Therefore, we have a 'chicken and egg' scenario.

All kinds of things can produce a leaky gut. For example, when I used to train for ultra-marathons I may have been doing some real damage to my gut, not just my joints. Antibiotic use, medications for acid reflux, non-steroidal anti-inflammatories (NSAIDs), stress and a diet high in gluten and processed foods are other known contributors to compromised gut lining integrity.[133] Gluten is implicated because it triggers the release of zonulin, a protein recognized as being a mediator of intestinal permeability.[134]

To repair a leaky gut

Firstly, focus on your diet and remove all inflammatory foods such as gluten, sugar, dairy, refined oils and artificial sweeteners. Eat nutrient-dense foods such as fruits, vegetables, lean organic meats, gluten-free grains like buckwheat, healthy fats, fermented vegetables and nuts.

Bone broth is gold when it comes to repairing your gut because it contains collagen. The intestinal wall is made up of microscopic folds referred to as villi, and these are built from collagen. Also, the amino acids in collagen support tissue growth in the gut. The most abundant amino acids in collagen, proline and glycine can help to heal a damaged intestinal wall.

The vagus nerve

The vagus nerve is smack bang in the middle of the gut–brain axis and is incredibly important.[135] A recent study involved administering *lactobacillus reuteri* — a probiotic bacteria that is found in the gastrointestinal tract, urinary tract, skin and breast milk of humans and other mammals[136] — to mice with autism-like behaviours via the vagus nerve.[137] The authors had discovered in 2016 that the offspring of mice fed a high-fat diet had a reduction in the bacterial species *L. reuteri,* and this led to social deficits (perhaps applicable to us socially awkward humans too). Importantly, in this study, when restored, the *L. reuteri* reversed the social deficits.

The researchers then severed the vagus nerve in the mice, and as a result *L. reuteri* had no effect on social behaviour in autistic mice. This indicates that the vagus nerve sends microbiome messages from the depths of the gut to the heights of our brain. It's like an old-school telephone … messages along a phone line.

The vagus nerve also plays a role in reducing inflammation. It operates a network of fibres that surround our organs, and relays information regarding the presence of inflammatory mediators. It acts like a spy that passes information about inflammation to the brain, so then the brain can respond and regulate the body's immune response.

~

Looking after your vagus nerve

Balancing the microbiome can increase the tone of the vagus nerve, which then increases parasympathetic nervous-system activation and calms us.

We can also increase the tone of the vagus nerve through meditation, humming or gargling, or slow, rhythmic, diaphragmatic breathing.

Increasing tone is associated with reduced inflammation, increased emotional regulation and reduced anxiety — and who doesn't want that, right?

Looking after the vagus nerve is important for gut-brain axis and will assist in the reduction of inflammation for a healthy mind.

Caring for our microbiome

Dramatic changes in our food system have negatively influenced the diverse and plentiful communities of bacteria in our gut. Antibiotics also significantly decrease the diversity of bacteria as they kill off many beneficial bacteria, as well as pathogenic strains.[138] Recent research has suggested that childhood illness and hospitalisation leaves us at greater risk of a disordered mind,[139] due to the antibiotics administered to fight off infection.

While antibiotics serve a purpose and save lives, it is important to work with your health practitioner and ask questions. Ask whether the antibiotics prescribed are broad spectrum as opposed to a narrow spectrum. If prescribed a broad-spectrum antibiotic such as amoxicillin, enquire whether a narrow-spectrum antibiotic would be effective. A narrow-spectrum drug such as a penicillin G (an older type of penicillin) is less likely to decimate all good bacteria as well as bad.

The news isn't all bad. Though antibiotics are linked to deprivation of gut bacteria, the composition and function of gut bacteria can recover after short-term antibiotic treatment in healthy people. But, more bad news: after six months, nine common beneficial bacterial species remain wiped out.[140]

If you have no choice but to take a course of antibiotics, make sure you also take a probiotic, because the antibiotic will almost certainly wipe out the good bacteria. Most likely you won't have enough good guys to keep yeast growth under control, which is why thrush is so common after antibiotics. Candida albicans is a yeast that is normally kept under control by bacteria (lactobacillus in particular) in the gut, and it grows like crazy when left to its own devices. To keep candida at bay after antibiotics, cut sugar (yeast loves sugar — in fact more often than not when we crave sugar, the nasty guys in our gut are calling the shots!), adopt a moderately low carbohydrate diet, and take herbal antifungal supplements such as oregano.

Plenty of probiotic supplements on the market can make choosing the right one quite confusing. Studies suggest that a portion of the population are actually resistant to probiotics — in other words, the bacteria they are ingesting do not manage to stay and recolonize their gut.[141] These findings argue that, like everything, rather than a universal approach or prescription, the use of probiotics should be tailored to the needs of each individual. This would mean an individual gut microbiome analysis performed by a health practitioner.

Also, the road leading to the gut can be a treacherous one. Stomach acid will kill many probiotic strains, and that's only if they manage to survive the microencapsulation and freeze-drying process. In saying that, probiotics do exert an effect by shifting gut community dynamics, and influencing the immune system while in transit.[142] A multitude of findings show that the ingestion of probiotics has benefits for anxiety, depression and many other ailments.[143]

Spore-based probiotics have a powerful impact on gut microbe diversity, because they can survive the stomach acid and then also survive in the external environment because they form a protective shell — an endospore — to protect themselves.[144] They then find bad bacteria and kill them off while feeding the good-guys prebiotics. Spore-based probiotics are generally found in the soil and that's why we should be out playing in the dirt more.

A recent study showed that when dietary endotoxemia is present — producing an inflammatory response in the body after a high fat/high calorie meal (which is common in Western countries), a spore-based probiotic is very effective.[145] The study involved 30 days of spore-based supplementation given to those who respond with elevated inflammatory markers after a high-fat meal; in this case a thin-crust cheese pizza. After 30 days of supplementation, diet-induced endotoxin and inflammation after the meal was significantly reduced.

A study in the *Brain, Behavior and Immunity* journal investigated whether changing the array of bacteria in the gut through probiotic supplements had a positive effect on mood. The study provided the probiotic to twenty healthy individuals, none of whom had a mood disorder, over a four-week period. A similar group of twenty non-depressed individuals received a placebo over the same period. At the conclusion of the study, both groups were tested to determine their reactivity, in terms of depression. It was concluded that there was a significant reduction in the degree change, in terms of cognitive reactivity to sad mood, in the group receiving the probiotic when compared to placebo.[146] What really stood out as a highlight of this study is that the probiotic exerted the strongest effects for reducing rumination and aggressive thoughts.

Several other studies have reported that when people take probiotics their anxiety levels, perception of stress and mental outlook improve, compared with those who don't take a probiotic.[147] Probiotics need food too, which is why prebiotics are vitally important. Prebiotics enable the probiotics to carry out their work. You can obtain prebiotics from insoluble fibre in your diet.

~

Prebiotics

Prebiotics are the three-course meal your healthy gut microbiome want to dine on. The best way to get prebiotics is to drive up your intake of soluble fibre-rich foods such as chicory root, dandelion greens, garlic, leeks, onions, sweet potatoes and asparagus.

Along with prebiotic foods, adding probiotics to your daily eating plan is important. Probiotics are designed to benefit the gut by adding good bacteria, which will leave less space for bad bacteria, thus enabling the whole community of the gut microbiome to produce beneficial compounds for the rest of the body to use.

Adding foods such as sauerkraut, kimchi, kefir and kombucha into your diet will naturally improve microbe diversity. As mentioned earlier, taking a probiotic supplement is also beneficial.

So, we have covered the ways the food system has changed, and the devastating impact it has had on our mind's health. Also, we know that the link between food, gut health and a well mind is strong and very important. Next we will explore some supplements and nutrients that can be beneficial for a well mind.

~

Gut microbiome testing

There are a number of companies in Australia, and internationally, that offer microbiome testing kits delivered to your home. In most cases you take a swab of stool and send it away to the designated laboratory for an in-depth analysis.

You should receive a comprehensive list of the beneficial and pathogenic microbes in your gut as well as relative abundance of each. You will receive information about diversity of gut microbes, and dietary suggestions to support gut health, and you should also receive information on any yeast overgrowth or pathogens present.

I feel it important to point out that this kind of commercial testing is not backed by science. One criticism is that samples should be whole stools because the core bacteria sit right in the middle of the stool, so a swab will not give a comprehensive insight into your microbiome. Another point is that these tests may give nutritional advice based on what bacteria is in abundance. An example is if we find that we have small amounts of bacteria responsible for converting glucosinolates found in cruciferous vegetables, we may be informed that we should reduce intake of cruciferous vegetables. This goes against everything we know concerning the health benefits of cruciferous vegetables such as broccoli, Brussels sprouts, cabbage, et cetera.

Our gut microbiome is not static and everyone has different levels of microbes at different times. So, if you do invest in one of these testing kits please approach the results with caution (or seek the support of a professional functional medicine practitioner).

Feed and supplement

As I began to take more care with what I put into my body I started to notice changes in my mental processes. I became much calmer and less reactive, and physical symptoms of anxiety lessened. My thoughts have slowed enough that I can stop, think and then react. The busy, loud, commotion in my head visits less frequently, and I am unmedicated. I have always suffered from what I can only describe as tickles on the inside of my abdomen, since I was a teen. I would just squirm and want to scratch my insides. Admittedly I still suffer occasionally, but far less than before.

Over the past couple of years I have been experimenting more with supplements and specific nutrients, and to date there have been good results. I feel that I have exceeded simply 'managing' my mental pain now and I feel that I am thriving (most of the time).

In this chapter I will list the nutrients important for mind health (some of which I have already mentioned), and food sources of those nutrients if applicable. Then, if you feel that you won't obtain adequate intake from food sources, a supplement may be beneficial. In saying that, it is important to view this information as a guide only. Always consult a qualified medical professional before embarking on any new diet or supplement program.

We tend to think of supplements in terms of the physical benefits that they may bring, rather than benefits for the mind. But nutritional deficiencies can masquerade as depression and anxiety, and in some cases even psychosis.[148] The current paradigm of obtaining all of our nutrients from food needs to be re-evaluated, because evidence suggests that a significant number of people suffering with an unwell mind have nutrient deficiencies, and therefore do not obtain adequate nutrition from their diet.[149] For example, in a study looking at vitamin D deficiency in psychiatric patients, 272 patients out of 290 were found to be deficient in vitamin D.[150]

Certain industrialized farming techniques are reported to have depleted the soil of essential nutrients, though little evidence supports this case, in Australia at least.[151] Regardless, it is a consideration, and other factors also impact our nutrient intake.

Our modern-day exposure to high amounts of toxins affects our ability to absorb some nutrients. Also important is that eating grain-fed animals is vastly different from grass-fed, in terms of nutritional status. Grain-fed animals are low in micronutrients, minerals and vitamins.[152]

And of course stress, gut dysbiosis and a high processed-food intake which will reduce nutritional density, leaving our mind starved for nutrients.

Following is a list of nutrients and supplements to consider on your journey to a well mind. Importantly, supplementation is not an excuse to eat poorly. When we consider the low absorption of nutrients from foods, and take into consideration other factors that affect our ability to utilize nutrients from foods, supplementation is merely that. We still need nourishment from a healthy diet. First up is omega-3 fatty acids — yes, I know we touched on this earlier, but it's so important, I need to re-iterate.

Omega-3 fatty acids

We know that omega-3 fatty acid supplementation is recognized as promoting brain and mind health. Omega-3 fatty acids regulate the production of neurotrophic factors, which impact the growth of new brain cells and effect emotional regulation.[153] These fatty acids can also influence gene expression in the brain.[154] But the number one important point to make is that omega-3 fatty acids are anti-inflammatory; and again — reduced inflammation improves the health of our mind.

Omega-3 fatty acids are made up of the long chain fatty acids docosahexaenoic acid, or DHA, and eicosapentaenoic acid, EPA, found in seafood. Together they reduce inflammation. There is some evidence that DHA is more crucial because it's the most prevalent fatty acid found in our brain, but both are important. Alpha-linolenic acid (ALA) is found in plants such as flaxseed and are short chain fatty acids. You have to eat more of these to get the same benefits as you get from consuming fish and shellfish.

Only one study, the VITamin D and OmegA-3 TriaL-Depression Endpoint Prevention (VITAL-DEP), has compared dosage, and 1 gram per day showed the greatest mood improvement.[155] People also ask what is best: fish oil or krill oil? A 2013 study published in *Lipids in Health and Disease*, reported that krill oil was more effective in a four-week trial,[156] but a similar study published in the same journal in 2015 showed no difference over four weeks.[157] Krill are bottom-feeding crustaceans, and thus krill oil can often be contaminated with pollutants in the ocean. In fact, Amanda

Dawson and colleagues highlighted that krill ingest microplastics, and the microplastics remain in the tissue of the krill, therefore will be consumed by any creature eating the krill.[158]

There are also suggestions that obtaining omega-3 EPA and DHA from fish oil is not the best way to go. Yes, we should eat wild-caught fatty fish a few times a week, but in terms of supplements, cod liver oil may be a better choice, due to its impressive vitamin A and D profile (vitamin D being important for a well mind).

B vitamins

Vitamin B1 (thiamine), B3 (niacin), B6, B9 (folate) and B12 have all been linked to the health of our mind. B group vitamins are cofactors for key enzymes that control balance of neurotransmitters (chemical messengers). A cofactor helps speed up chemical reactions (or the conversion of one chemical to another). Serotonin (5-HT) is produced from 5-HTP by the addition of a methyl group (carboxylase). This is similar for the conversion of adrenaline from noradrenaline. All of the complex neurotransmitter conversion is dependent on vitamin B12, 6 and folate. Although this seems complex, the important point is that B vitamins are crucial for the balance of neurotransmitters that play a role in attaining a well mind.

Some studies have shown that vitamin B deficiency can be mistaken for a mood disorder, and supplementation with folate and B12 can improve depression.[159] One study, published in the *American Journal of Psychiatry*, reported that in a cohort of disabled women aged sixty-five and over, those deficient in B12 had a two-fold increase in severe depression than those non deficient.[160] The cross-sectional nature of the study makes it difficult to determine cause and effect; however, we need to be aware of a link between vitamin B12 deficiency and depression.

In his book *Nutrient Power: Heal your biochemistry and heal your brain*, William J Walsh[161] discusses symptoms of folate deficiency depression. This is important because it illustrates that a nutrient deficiency can masquerade as mental illness. He lists some symptoms as: low libido, sleep disorders, and anxiety and panic tendencies.

Vitamin B rich foods

Foods that contain thiamine:

- nutritional yeast
- sunflower seeds
- macadamia nuts
- seaweed
- organic edamame
- broad beans
- beef liver
- Brussels sprouts
- asparagus.

Foods that contain B6:

- turkey
- grass-fed beef
- tuna
- avocado
- chicken breast
- sunflower seeds
- sesame seeds
- spinach
- pistachio nuts
- chickpeas.

Foods that contain niacin:

- chicken
- liver
- turkey
- tuna
- salmon
- sardines
- grass-fed beef
- sunflower seeds
- green peas
- brown rice
- mushrooms
- avocado
- sweet potato.

Foods that contain folate:

- beef liver
- spinach and kale
- asparagus
- eggs
- beets
- Brussels sprouts
- broccoli.

Foods high in B12:

- beef liver
- clams
- mussels
- sardines
- salmon
- mackerel
- tuna
- Greek yoghurt
- cheese
- grass-fed beef
- eggs.

If you have symptoms of depression, anxiety or brain fog, get your doctor to check for vitamin B deficiency.

Vitamin D

Evidence suggests that symptoms of vitamin D deficiency can also be confused with mental illness. Recently Canadian researchers conducted a systematic review — their analysis of fourteen studies revealed an association between vitamin D levels and depression. It seems that low levels of vitamin D corresponded to symptoms of depression, and increased odds for depression.[162] And there are many studies linking vitamin D supplementation with improved mood and wellbeing.[163] In one study contained in the *Journal of Preventative Medicine*, women receiving 50,000 IU vitamin D3 had improved mood status and decreased inflammation.[164] Vitamin D is available in two forms: vitamin D2 (ergocalciferol) and vitamin D3 (cholecalciferol). Vitamin D3 is considered superior because it is almost twice as effective at increasing D levels in the blood.[165] Therefore, taking a vitamin D3 supplement is recommended; especially in our 'sun smart' culture. Before you discuss mood disorders with your GP, please get your vitamin D levels checked.

How to get Vitamin D

Foods that contain vitamin D3:

- salmon
- mackerel
- tuna
- beef liver
- cod liver oil
- oysters
- eggs.

Sun exposure: Getting out in the sun for 10-15 minutes a couple of times a week is generally enough. However, older adults and those with darker skin may not synthesize vitamin D well. It is interesting that our diligent use of sunblock and our avoidance of the sun have coincided with an increase in reported mental illness.

Magnesium

Magnesium is essential for optimal brain function, and deficiency has been linked to depression, anxiety and other mood disorders.

In fact, a large study published in the *American Board of Family Medicine* reported that those with low magnesium intake had a greater than 50 percent increase in symptoms of depression over three years.[166] And in a recent meta-analysis including eleven studies looking at the relationship between magnesium and depression, those who had the lowest intake of magnesium were 81 percent more likely to be depressed than those with the highest intake.[167] In 2017 a randomized clinical trial found that supplementation with magnesium citrate led to significant improvements in depression and anxiety regardless of age, gender or severity of depression.[168]

Although plenty of evidence suggests that magnesium may contribute to a well mind,[169] some flaws exist in the research, such as cross-sectional study design and possible reverse causality (for example, is poor dietary intake of magnesium a result of poor mental health, or does it contribute to poor mental health?); and so more research is required. However, there is evidence linking low levels of magnesium in the blood with chronic inflammation, so eating magnesium-rich foods or taking a supplement is highly recommended.[170]

Agricultural practices that deplete the soil of magnesium, as well as food processing and increased levels of stress will likely render us deficient in magnesium.[171] Also, leaky gut can cause malabsorption of minerals such as magnesium.[172]

Magnesium citrate, as you would expect, is magnesium with citrate, and it can have a laxative effect in some people. Magnesium glycinate has optimal bioavailability, and is the most popular form of magnesium for muscle relaxation.

The newest form of magnesium on the market, magnesium-L-threonate — considered a 'breakthrough' supplement — has great bioavailability and also the potential to improve cognitive functions.[173] A recent study using magnesium-L-threonate, demonstrated that twelve-week administration not only boosted performance on individual cognitive tests, but also reversed brain deterioration by more than nine years in older adults with cognitive impairment.[174]

Foods that contain magnesium:

- avocado
- figs
- spinach
- chard
- dark chocolate
- almonds
- pumpkin seeds
- black beans.

Zinc

Zinc is a nutrient that can modulate the brain and body's response to life stressors. Dietary zinc deficiency can result in depression-like symptoms, and generally, blood levels of zinc are lower in those suffering with mood disorders.[175] In fact, zinc is vitally important in the communication between neural networks. Research has confirmed that communication between neurons in the hippocampus (the area of the brain responsible for emotional regulation), is also reliant upon adequate levels of zinc.[176] Zinc is necessary for a healthy mind, and if you can't obtain adequate amounts from food, consider a supplement.

Foods high in zinc:

- grass-fed beef
- shellfish
- lentils
- pumpkin seeds
- hemp seeds
- cashews
- yoghurt
- shiitake mushrooms
- spinach
- avocado
- ricotta cheese
- chicken
- almonds.

Supplements

I want to reiterate, it is important that you speak to a medical practitioner before starting a new supplement or dietary regime.

N-Acetyl Cysteine (NAC)

N-Acetyl Cysteine (NAC) is one of the most impressive supplements I have come across, other than omega-3, for brain health. Research shows that it holds benefits for those with depression, anxiety, bipolar and obsessive compulsive disorder (OCD).[177]

NAC has been well reviewed for its antioxidant and anti-inflammatory actions.[178] It increases the production of glutathione, an important antioxidant that helps reduce free radical damage and plays a role in the detoxification of heavy metals and other harmful substances. The thing that intrigues me about glutathione is its implications for mental health due to its ability to lower oxidative stress; interestingly, those suffering mental health issues have lower levels of glutathione.

A systematic review suggests that favourable evidence supports NAC in the treatment of major depressive disorder, bipolar disorder, drug addiction, obsessive-compulsive disorder, autism, schizophrenia, Alzheimer's disease and certain forms of epilepsy (progressive myoclonic).[179] Also, the use of NAC in anxiety and attention deficit hyperactivity disorder (ADHD) has some supporting preliminary evidence, but requires larger studies to confirm.[180]

At the time of writing I have been taking NAC for approximately nine months and have had many comments on how calm and happy I seem. Now, there are many potential contributing factors, but I do feel that NAC is improving the health of my mind.

5-HTP

We make 5-Hydroxytryptophan (5-HTP) from the amino acid tryptophan. Then, 5-HTP is converted into serotonin and melatonin. And serotonin can contribute to a happy, healthy mind. Because 5-HTP is converted to melatonin it can aid sleep, which leads to reduced inflammation.

The studies to date on 5-HTP intake have been positive, but have included small sample sizes, and have sometimes lacked a control group.[181] It would appear that 5-HTP may have beneficial effects on mood, but good quality, randomized control trials are needed to confirm this.[182]

SAMe

S-adenosylmethionine (SAMe) is a chemical made naturally in the body, from methionine, an amino acid found in foods such as egg whites, wild-caught fish, oats and sesame seeds. It has been reported to regulate key functions in living cells. SAMe increases the rate of production of serotonin, and may stimulate production of dopamine and norepinephrine.[183] It has been shown to have anti-inflammatory effects, and therefore may be important in healing the mind.[184]

Abnormal levels of SAMe in the body have been observed in depression, which motivated researchers to investigate if SAMe may have beneficial effects for mood regulation, and it appears that it does.[185] It has also been reported that SAMe may be effective in drug treatment resistant patients (those who find that antidepressants and other drugs do not help).

Gamma-aminobutyric acid (GABA)

Gamma-aminobutyric acid (GABA) is an amino acid produced naturally in the brain and is believed to have anti-anxiety properties. GABA lowers the activity of neural cells in the brain and seems to be effective at moving the brain and the body into low gear. Because it inhibits neural activity, GABA is excellent for aiding sleep, reducing mental and physical stress, and creating overall Zen. Alcohol binds well to GABA receptors, which is why we feel relaxed when we drink.

A large study published in the journal *Amino Acids* researched the effects of 100 mg of GABA among a group of people who had recently undertaken a stressful mental task. Brainwaves slowed and mental stress was alleviated.[186] And another study from the *International Journal of Food Sciences and Nutrition*, conducted in 2009, found that eating chocolate containing 28 mg of GABA reduced stress in participants performing a problem-solving task.[187] And who wouldn't like a little stress reduction? Also, a small study reported recently that taking 300 mg of GABA an hour before retiring to bed helped sleep in comparison to a placebo. This tracked on to improvements being maintained four weeks after starting treatment.[188]

Ashwagandha

Ashwagandha (*Withania somnifera*) is a herb commonly used in Ayurveda, the traditional medicine of India. I am a big fan of ayurvedic medicine because its definition of health focuses on a healthy mind as well as a healthy body. Ayurveda encompasses the symbiotic relationship among the mind, body, soul, the senses and all of their workings.

The root of ashwagandha smells like a horse and it is believed it gives the strength and virility of a horse (in Sanskrit, *ashva* means 'horse' and *gandha* means 'smell').

This herb is what we refer to as an adaptogen, which means it is a substance that helps the body adapt to stress. It lowers cortisol levels, so it has potential to be very helpful for those prone to anxiety. Ashwagandha is also reported to increase immunity, improve sleep, improve concentration and increase libido.[189]

Numerous controlled human studies have shown that ashwagandha effectively reduces symptoms in people with stress and anxiety disorders.[190] In a 60-day study in 64 people with chronic stress, those who were taking ashwagandha reported a 69 percent average reduction in anxiety and insomnia, compared to 11 percent in the placebo group.[191] In another study, 88 percent of people who took ashwagandha reported a reduction in anxiety, compared to 50 percent of those who took a placebo.[192]

Some research indicates that ashwagandha may reduce depression and also have beneficial effects in those diagnosed with bipolar disorder and generalized anxiety disorder.[193] A 2015 study published in the *Journal of Ethnopharmocology* demonstrated that ashwagandha blocks the stress pathway in the brains of rats by regulating chemical signalling in the nervous system and activating GABA.[194] Three controlled trials (2000, 2009 and 2012) reported that ashwagandha supplementation can reduce stress and anxiety symptoms in people with related disorders.[195]

Brahmi

Brahmi (*Bacopa monnieri*) is a small creeping herb with an ancient reputation for reducing stress. Like ashwagandha, brahmi is an adaptogen. It is believed this herb increases serotonin levels in the brain that help the mind keep calm and give relief from anxiety and nervousness. There is evidence that brahmi influences the brain's ability to regenerate brain tissue.[196] However, there isn't enough evidence in human studies to make concrete claims regarding benefits for inflammation, but in animal studies brahmi's impressive anti-inflammatory actions have been demonstrated.[197]

Lemon balm

Lemon balm (*Melissa officinalis*) is member of the mint family. It smells amazing and has been used throughout history to ease the nervous system. A number of studies have suggested that lemon balm can also help alleviate stress and induce calm.[198]

One compelling study suggests that lemon balm drinks (a sweetened water-based drink containing 0.3 grams of lemon balm extract) can improve mood and also help cognitive performance.[199]

~

So, now we have explored some supplements and nutrients that will support a well mind. Other factors such as technology use, sleep, stress and exercise also have an effect on the health of our mind, and we will dive into those next.

CHAPTER 9:

Protect
Your Mind

'Technology has solved old economic problems by giving us new psychological problems. The internet has not just open-sourced information, it has also open-sourced insecurity, self-doubt, and shame.'

Mark Manson

Sarah wakes up to her alarm at 6 a.m. and hits snooze, rolls over and sleeps for another 30 minutes. She was up until 12.30 a.m., comforting herself with a Netflix binge after a tough day at work.

Still sleepy, she reaches for her phone and goes straight to Instagram, smiling as she sees six new followers, and seventeen likes on a post she painstakingly put together before climbing into bed. After a quick look through all the Instagram stories, she switches over to Facebook and is alarmed to see no likes on a post from 9 p.m.

Her mind is in a spin: 'Surely Nikki was on Facebook and she always likes my posts … and Aunty Joan is obsessed with social media, so she must have seen it?' she thinks to herself. She goes to the post and checks again. 'That was such a silly thing to write — did I spell transparency right?' she frantically thinks. 'And look at what I'm wearing … Maybe I'll delete it — I'm such a loser.'

Sarah catches a glimpse of the time while checking her post again. 'Oh no, it's almost seven-thirty, and I haven't exercised or done my morning meditation yet again … Okay, well, I'll just take a selfie on the way to work with a coffee in my hand, and rocking my new green dress, and hopefully no one will notice the terrible response rate to my post last night.'

Not sure if you can relate … I certainly can.

This is the world we live in, my friends. Sarah was hooked on the dopamine reward that we receive with social engagement; and Facebook and other social media tick all the boxes for the addictive hit.[200] When she didn't get the hit of dopamine, panic set in and she spent precious time worrying about it.

Now, with the stress of not getting enough likes on your post aside, when was the last time you sat on a train and just looked out the window? When was the last time you sat in a cafe waiting for a friend without checking your social media accounts, email, or indulging in a little swiping right or left? Been a while, hey?

Hooked on our screens

We may be more connected, but since the advent of smart phones and social media we have reduced face-to-face interaction, and it can impact our mental health. We are becoming more disconnected from self and others, and is it any wonder when we are intent on using our time to stare at a screen? Research coming out from the University of Pittsburgh School of Medicine involving more than 1700 young adults using social media platforms reports that those who spent more than two hours a day interacting with social media are twice as likely to experience social isolation than those spending less than 30 minutes.[201]

Even Facebook agrees that social media can be bad for our minds.[202] Hello! Have you had a look around a restaurant recently and observed couples, families and friends all with their heads stuck in their phones? I have even glimpsed people in the movie cinema checking their phone at a key moment in the plot — after they have spent good money to see the movie. We can access everything on our smart phones: food, social interaction, relationships, sex, social approval, the list goes on. And so, we are hooked on a screen.

Research suggests that pre-teens and teens using smartphones have trouble focusing, and symptoms of disorders such as ADHD manifest.[203] Further to that, there is a link between depression and smartphone/social media use.[204] Although we can't state for sure that depression is a direct result of excessive technology use, there is strong argument that too much time spent on devices is a contributing factor. For example, the fast pace of the internet means information flies at us at the click of a mouse, which can be overwhelming and, consequently, depressing. We can lose touch with the real world and real people, and because we are offered instant gratification online, it is sometimes easier to stay online, rather than get out among other people. And this leaves us with a feeling of disconnect.[205]

And it's not only disconnect associated with excessive use of technology that is problematic: too much time spent in the company of devices breeds stress.

In America, 65 percent of adults admit that they constantly check personal email; 52 percent and 44 percent say the same about texts and social media respectively; and 28 percent (of those employed) report the same about their work email. Those who are constant checkers are more likely to say that this habit is a stressful aspect of technology.[206] In other words, checking our phone (this includes Instagram scrolling and Facebook surfing) is making us stressed and miserable.

Our reliance on a screen to avert the awkward feeling of having nothing to do, or using our phone to avoid the lonely boredom of waiting for a tardy friend to arrive, isn't the real problem. Nor is the hit to our self-esteem when our post doesn't receive the accolades that we thought it would. No, the real problem is the social isolation and addiction that can strike us all.

This is a great example of an oxymoron: 'social' and 'media'. We were led to believe that social media would open up our world socially, but the opposite is true. A recent study from the *American Journal of Preventative Medicine* has highlighted that those who use social media the most actually feel more socially isolated.[207]

It's addictive

Everyone knows it's damaging, and even Prince Harry (who reached a million followers on social media in record time) stated that social media is more addictive than alcohol and drugs, and therefore is more dangerous. Research has indicated that there is a link between social media and depression,[208] anxiety,[209] suicide risk[210] and sleep disruption,[211] and there aren't many of us out there now without a social media account.

The magnetic pull of social media is real, thanks to dopamine and oxytocin (our love drugs). Tweeting for ten minutes can raise oxytocin levels in the blood as much as 13 percent, and this chemical increases during social bonding, and also sex. As mentioned, dopamine is addictive and motivates you to seek, and then you get rewarded, which makes you seek more. So, it becomes increasingly difficult to stop checking likes and followers on social media, and to stop looking at your phone to see if you have new messages.[212]

Technology seductively sucks up our time and does not return it, and we therefore have less time for face-to-face interaction. And we are hooked.

Everyone else is happy?

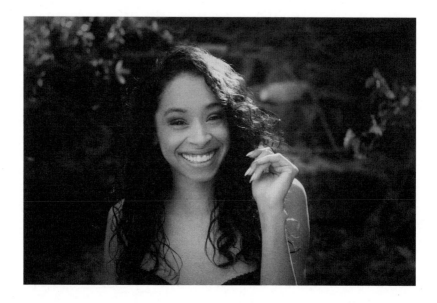

The woman in this photo looks happy, doesn't she? But she is merely posing for a photo, so how happy is she really?

I have smiled brightly for many photos while feeling like I was dying inside. And I judge the photo by how big my grin is rather than how I am feeling at the time. Often, when we are mentally well, a smile is contagious and warms us; however, it can take a toll when our minds aren't doing so well. We see smiling faces on our social media feeds daily and it can prompt us to dwell on any discomfort and unhappiness we may experience. We should remember that, like the woman here in the photo, most smiling happy faces are impermanent and primed for the camera lens in that moment.

It's a subconscious process when we measure how we stack up against others, and if we aren't feeling robust and content in our lives, it can lead to a devastating sense of failure and despair. We see everyone posting their holiday to the Greek islands, their new car, their slim body, their happy relationship, their great social life, their perfect skin (urgh), and we believe that everyone else is happy — except us. Of course this is not the case, but that's what we see.

Several studies point to an association between social comparison or envy, depression and poor mental health.[213] Facebook is now fifteen years old and it certainly hasn't improved the wellness of our mind — that I'm aware of, anyway. The irony is that we are all performing at our perfect 'front stage' self on social media (have you ever watched a couple of teens agonize over the perfect background and pose for a selfie — it can literally take 45 minutes) while feeling bad about ourselves when we see everyone else at their perfect best.

To be fair, we did have social envy, loneliness, predisposition to comparison disorders and a longing for distraction before social media: these are in part what makes us human. But we need some balance or it becomes a problem.

So, other than deleting our social media accounts, what can we do to mitigate the impact that social media has on the wellbeing of our mind? Here are some tips that may help.

~

Reduce social media time

- Remove the apps from your phone. Not having such easy access to Instagram, Facebook and Twitter makes it less likely that you will check in as often.

- Stop comparing. Remind yourself that everyone has ups and downs and that what you see is just a post of someone in their 'onstage self'.

- Keep your phone out of your bedroom. Checking your feed before you sleep is a sure-fire way of ensuring your sleep quality is not optimal. Waking up and checking your phone is also not conducive to a healthy mind. Start your day with gratitude, meditation and exercise — not a Facebook scroll. Allowing social media into the bedroom also impacts sex and healthy relationships.

- Unfollow accounts that feed into unhealthy thoughts. For example, if you are feeling bad about your body it may be unwise to follow someone who is posting hot bikini shots all over the place. Take time to reflect on why this account is triggering negative emotions.

- Set limits on the time spent on these apps. Set a timer if need be. The time spent scrolling through your feed is time that you can never get back, and unless it is contributing to your health and wellbeing in some way, try to reduce exposure.

- Take regular breaks from social media. A feeling of freedom will accompany ditching the phone. Imagine how much time you could save having a break, and then reinvest that time into catching up with people in person.

As mentioned, the frequent use of devices has led to us feeling more socially isolated, and this can translate to loneliness. Loneliness is a growing problem globally and in Australia one in four people report feeling lonely each week, according to the Australian Loneliness report. [214]

Loneliness

During my adult years I have cancelled too many social engagements to mention because I didn't have the energy or capacity to engage with others in a suitable manner. Sometimes the 'normal' way people converse is too much for me to bear: I long for what I believe are 'real' conversations filled with passion, colour and meaning. Only problem is, often I don't even know what that means.

The fruits of poor mental health have cumulated in a sense of loneliness for me on a multitude of occasions. People have abandoned me, criticized me, even been afraid of me. I can understand why, but understanding doesn't alleviate the pain associated with feeling lonely.

Loneliness is devastating. Even Charlie Brown knew this, when he visited Lucy's psychiatric booth and asked if she could cure loneliness. Lucy replied that for a nickel she could cure anything, and so Charlie Brown expanded and described real loneliness as 'deep-down, black, bottom-of-the-well, no-hope, end-of-the-world, what's-the-use loneliness'.[215] It's a great description of the emptiness of feeling lonely.

We crave connection with others. Indeed, a review published in the *Annals of Behavioural Medicine*, looking at physical and mental consequences of loneliness, suggests that social isolation can have a terrible effect on our mind and can detrimentally influence mood, perspective and the ability to cope with stress.[216]

Satisfying social interaction is vital for the wellbeing of the mind, and one consequence of loneliness is reduced capacity for self-regulation. This means that when lonely we have trouble regulating thoughts, feelings and behaviour, so then we may have diminished capacity to regulate lifestyle behaviours such as sleep, physical activity and other health-promoting activities.[217]

One strategy is to understand and acknowledge your loneliness — by making the effort to talk to others about feeling lonely we are likely to discover that they often feel the same.

~

How to guard against loneliness

- Disconnect from social media, which gives false perceptions and can create a feeling of loneliness.

- Understand that loneliness is a feeling and is not permanent.

- Get out of your comfort zone and try something new. For example, take up surfing, or join a hiking group.

- Even when your loneliness is telling you that no one cares, reach out to family and friends and initiate face time and conversation.

- Join a club to meet others with shared interests.

- Volunteer with a charity or an organisation where you can help others.

- Get to know your neighbours. This may also help another person who is feeling lonely and disconnected.

~

Host a 'well mind' dinner

Get a few people together for a 'well mind' night. Prepare a meal that is both anti-inflammatory and nourishing for your mind, and share tips on what you are doing to maintain a well mind. Encourage each other to make lifestyle changes for the health and wellbeing of your minds and bodies. Make it a ritual and aim for at least one combined dinner and encouragement session a month.

Stress

Chronic stress has been part of my life for as long as I can remember. During early manic episodes I often decimated my credit card and left a trail of carnage behind me. I would swing back and forth according to my impulses. The exhilaration of participating in dangerous activities was too much to resist, but the stress of dealing with what was waiting for me when I came back down was significant. Unfortunately, stress is also a trigger for a manic or depressive episode, so it's a bit of a merry go round.

In periods of mania I would easily work fourteen-hour days; and even in earlier years when at home looking after my babies I was go, go, go, always fuelled by a stream of cortisol and adrenaline. It didn't take long before I was fatigued, dizzy, suffering heart palpitations, unable to concentrate and experiencing panic attacks.

It has been a work in progress for me to manage my stress. My mother gave me a wonderful compliment recently when she told me how in earlier years I was like a fragile piece of china that had the appearance of shattering into little pieces at any given time — so much so that she was afraid to hug me — but lately she has seen a significant change in my disposition. It feels amazing when others notice the improvements within me. I still suffer from stress: just far less often.

So many of us are stressed. We are constantly on call (or constantly checking devices). Back in our ancestral, hunter–gatherer days our sympathetic nervous system (fight-or-flight) response only activated when we came across a lion while out on a daily jog to catch food. Then, we would use the secreted adrenaline and cortisol, which would increase our heart rate and reduce our autonomic nervous system functions, to give us bursts of energy to get the hell out of there.

Once we had outrun that killer lion, we would gradually calm down and resume as normal (well, perhaps resume a little apprehensively). The problem is that we aren't just running away from the lion now; we are meeting deadlines, dealing with family problems, financial problems, work problems, relationship problems, teenage problems and all kinds of other life problems. Stress is chronic and long lasting.

Emily's story

Emily had a high-pressure job, and put herself under additional pressure trying to keep up with friends and family, rarely saying no in case she offended someone. Weekends were gobbled up with the overflow of work tasks that she couldn't manage during the week. At the end of an incredibly tough couple of months, she reported gastrointestinal issues, fatigue, insomnia and depression and didn't know where to turn.

Emily's situation is common in the 21st century, and this kind of ongoing stress has terrible effects on our mind.

Unfortunately Emily did 'burn out' and became seriously unwell. She was diagnosed with Hashimoto's disease, an autoimmune disease characterized by slowed thyroid hormone production. Because the adrenal glands that produce our stress hormones also produce hormones that regulate other major metabolic processes, such as thyroid hormone production and distribution, chronic stress can create havoc on our physiology. Problems with the thyroid gland can often manifest as depression and anxiety.[218]

Emily had to take drastic action. First she took some of her accrued holiday leave and focused on deleting any feelings of guilt about taking this unplanned leave, because she knew it was much needed. She then embarked on getting her health back and reducing chronic stress.

She took a month away from all social media and reduced time in front of a screen. Emily used this time to begin a meditation practice and spent time outdoors walking in nature.

Emily consulted a nutritionist, and had a gut microbiome test to assess the diversity of microbes in her gut. She cut back on caffeine and alcohol consumption and reduced processed foods and refined sugar because these feed nervous anxiety and depression.

Emily also used this time to visit with family and friends and re-evaluate her work–life balance. She made a commitment to only work Monday through Friday and to never let work creep into her weekends. She also stayed abreast of employment opportunities that were more flexible and less demanding than her current position.

Stress affects our nervous system significantly. Back in our hunter–gatherer days we didn't have the artificial light or the sensory stimulation that we have now, both of which impact sleep quality and stress levels. Today's influx of information, and changes to our community structure encountered throughout history have come in a huge rush. Humans simply haven't had time to evolve far from the safeguards in place to ensure our survival.

Busy, busy, busy

How on earth can we be calm and content when we can't focus? Most of us check our smart phones every twelve minutes (yes, that is a reported statistic),[219] and our focus is interrupted with email notifications all day. Our minds are all over the place, and consequently we have lost our ability to focus for long periods of time.[220] How can we find meaning and purpose in our lives when goldfish have longer attention spans than we do?

Being busy these days is often a badge of honour. I rarely have a conversation where I am asked, or ask, 'How are you?' without the answer including the word 'busy'. As a result we are all exceptional at multitasking. A study published in the journal *PLoS ONE* looked at the amount of time people spent on multiple devices (i.e., texting while watching TV), and then took MRI scans of their brains. They reported that high multitaskers had less brain density in the anterior cingulate cortex, a region responsible for empathy, as well as cognitive and emotional control.[221]

So, multitasking hurts our brains. And we are multitasking from the time we wake up — checking phones while watching TV, reading email while finishing a review — until we go to sleep. Our calendars are so full we can't comprehend not doing three things at once; we exist in a constant state of alertness and stress. And it is not conducive to a healthy and calm mind.

Although my pathology reared its head long before I had access to smartphones or social media, I can reflect that I had not experienced symptoms of a panic attack before I started using technology. Waking up at 5 a.m. and checking my email, to find that my inbox was full, is an early morning blast of cortisol to start the day.

Also, society pressures us to do everything, and do it exceptionally well, without help. Somewhere along the way we have lost track of what is important, and have adopted the inclination to measure our self-worth against others, or what society deems as successful.

As alluded to earlier I once believed I could be Wonder Woman. Clean and tidy home, with healthy meals cooked every evening. Check. Complete my PhD and make enough money to pay the mortgage. Check. Run 10–15 kilometres daily. Check. Make time to catch up with friends. Check. Maintain busy career and meet KPIs. Check. Head for burnout and mental breakdown. Check. There is no room to take care of the health of our mind when we are striving to excel on so many levels. Nor when we try to be everything to everyone.

It may been seen as presumptuous to state that we are more stressed than those who came before us. Past generations had to contend with war, plague and poverty. Mark Jackson, in his article 'The stress of life: A modern complaint?'[222] makes reference to an article in *The Times*, published in 1872, that suggested that rising death rates from heart disease were the 'unavoidable result of the great mental strain and hurried excitement' generated by steam and electricity, overcrowded communities, and the relentless and exhausting struggle for existence. So, we were stressed back then too.

Although the stress felt may be comparable, I argue that the 21st century offers a chronic stress that is difficult to escape, and so therefore is more deleterious. We have so much choice now in everything, and if we are prone to even a hint of anxiety, the abundance of choice is bound to cause friction within our mind. Supermarket shelves are packed with choice when compared to 60–70 years ago; in fact, the number of items on Australian supermarket shelves has more than doubled in just the past twenty years. The choice in entertainment is vast. My husband and I often sit scrolling through programs on Netflix, only to give up through choice overload.

In comparison to our grandparents we sit in traffic for longer, are surrounded by noise, and more people, and have so much to take in daily. There is pressure to be our best self, our most authentic self, all day, every day. And though technology can't be blamed for everything — and I'm not anti-technology — it has allowed us the freedom to work from anywhere 24/7, to be contacted at any time. The 40-hour work week becomes a distant memory. Ah the 'good ol' days'! Consequently, we are all so stressed.

Stress can manifest in many ways such as fatigue, digestive issues, thyroid issues, skin problems, headaches, chronic pain, decreased libido, rapid heartbeat, decreased appetite, hormonal imbalances, reduced immunity and more. If we want to get to a place where our minds are as healthy as they should be we need to learn to manage our stress well. We need to take back control and find ways to calm our nervous system.

Below are some strategies that work for me.

~

Stress reduction

- Make a point of not proclaiming 'busy' when asked how you are. In changing our mindset and realising that busy is not a badge of honour or a state to aspire to, we may prioritize being less busy.

- Take time to learn the kinds of situations that cause you stress. Be extra attentive to how your body feels when under stress, and take note of the things that affect you the most.

- Use a breathing technique, (see page 186). Breathe in through your nose for the count of four and out for the count of eight.

- Engage in regular exercise. (More on exercise soon.)

- Find someone you trust to open up with; expressing your feelings is important.

- Learn to delegate and to establish priorities.

- Learn meditation.

- Escape. Leave the stressful situation, go for a walk, read a book. If you can't physically leave, then escape with your mind. Daydream.

- Nourish your mind and body with nutrient-dense foods.

- Be kind to yourself and don't judge yourself for feeling overwhelmed.

- Focus on good sleep hygiene.

Sleep and exercise

I would lie in the darkness with energy surging through me and thoughts whizzing around my mind (I would sometimes see the thoughts in words running across the back of my eyelids as I squeezed them tightly shut). Tickles would travel around my torso: I wanted to scratch so badly to make them stop.

Eventually I would give up and escape my bed. Often it was to the exercise bike where I would pump my legs around and around for hours hoping to expend the torrent of energy racing around inside me. On occasion, ignoring any danger, I would leave the house in the early hours of the morning and go for a long run. I once arrived at work at 2 a.m. — I was of course the only person there apart from the cleaner who arrived three hours later. In my first marriage I managed to sneak out of bed often, but as I worked in the evening back then, sometimes I didn't even get to bed until 3 a.m. I now understand that sleep is as important as nutrition to keep my mind well, and I hold it in the highest regard.

Alan's story

Alan was hanging on by a thread. He suffered insomnia for five years, with sleep problems manifesting at the time of a stressful marriage breakdown. The toll on his mind was high. Alan had tried several prescription medications only to discontinue each due to either awful side effects or lack of efficacy. He was willing to try anything but felt so low he didn't hold much hope.

To keep functioning during the day Alan would knock back five or six cups of coffee. He also tried to nap wherever possible; even at his desk. He wasn't able to participate in any recreational activities — it was taking every ounce of energy just to function at work.

Alan tried to be in bed by 11.30 p.m., and often fell asleep within 30 minutes. He would wake two to three times every night and often get up to work on his laptop rather than waste the time staring at the ceiling. It was often 5 a.m. before he would go back to bed. His alarm was set at 6 a.m., however he would doze until 7.30 a.m.

Alan was desperate for help, and the first step was evaluation of his lifestyle and sleep hygiene.

After the evaluation I recommended that Alan reduce caffeine to one cup of black coffee consumed before lunch. He was advised to put his alarm out of reach so that he had to physically get out of bed to turn it off. Snoozing is a really unhealthy way to start the day, and he was encouraged to avoid going back to bed no matter how tired he was.

He was advised that when he couldn't sleep he should read and avoid screens (phone, computer, TV). Daily bed time had to change from 11.30 p.m. to 10 p.m. and he needed to quit his daily afternoon nap.

Because Alan scored high in stress and anxiety screenings he was advised to attend a meditation and relaxation course. He also committed to engage in some physical activity for at least 30 minutes each day.

Additionally, there was a psychophysiological aspect to Alan's insomnia. He had started to associate his bed with frustration due to many nights where he had wrestled with sleep there. It was advised that if he couldn't fall back to sleep twenty minutes after waking he go to another room and read until he felt sleepy enough to return to bed.

It took six weeks and Alan was a different man. At that stage it still took twenty minutes for him to fall asleep, so he also downloaded a relaxation app in the hope that he would drift off faster.

Alan kept his alarm in the bathroom where he could hear it, but had to get out of his bed to turn it off. He had only one cup of coffee in the morning and felt that his nervous system was benefitting greatly from this change. His stress levels reduced with regular exercise: exercise has a profound effect on the body and mind. It had taken effort to implement the changes, but they worked: the effort was worth it.

Changes to sleep over time

Think back to what life would have been like for our prehistoric ancestors. They would wake at dawn, literally at first light. They weren't out drinking and dancing at a club, or in front of a screen until 1 a.m., so no need for that decadent sleep in. Also, according to reports, they had segmented sleep where they would sleep in two blocks.[223] This makes sense, as for many hunter–gatherer tribes the requirement for someone to be awake during the night would be high, to protect the sleeping tribe. It is likely that everyone took turns to keep watch.

Additionally, Roger Ekirch, in his book *At Day's Close* discusses 'segmented sleep' later in history. There was the 'first sleep' until midnight, then the 'second sleep' until dawn. In between, we read or talked, had sex, smoked or meditated.[224] This nocturnal interlude ceased at some point in the 18th century when gas lamps were introduced. Around this time the Industrial Revolution introduced a 'work long and increase productivity' approach (smart, hey). Now we have shift work, artificial light, time-zone travel, all of which disrupt out basic circadian clock. Circadian rhythm disturbances are linked to inflammation, and inflammation is linked to poor health of our mind.

Sleep and our mind

Sometimes when I was flirting with mania, I enjoyed the super energy forcing through my mind. I would work, play and exercise: as far as I was concerned, sleep was a waste of time. 'I'll sleep when I'm dead,' I would proclaim. And then I would continue on the rapid incline up to the heights of pain, irritability and crazy until I started to plunge down the other side into the depths of depression and despair. When there, all I would want to do is sleep and hide in my bed.

Sleep is closely related to the health of our mind. Just recently a study published in the journal *Sleep*, involving 4175 teenagers, found that sleeping six hours or less a night increases risk of major depression.[225] In fact, because there are several correlations between sleep and mental illness, Russell Foster, Head of the Oxford Sleep and Circadian Neuroscience Institute stated, '*Sleep disruption is a very common feature of mental illness, yet despite its prevalence the clinical relevance is often overlooked and even when recognised, treatment options are limited.*'[226]

Sleep allows the brain to wash itself clean of waste (or, more specifically, proteins) that builds up between cells during the day. Some interesting research found that the brain cells of mice may actually shrink during sleep to accommodate the volume of liquid flowing in and out of the brain. As a result, there is an increase in the interstitial space, which appears to help clear out waste. The cells then expand once the mice wake up.[227]

Many of us are sleep deprived or have irregular sleep patterns, and the effects on our mind health are significant. As mentioned, I am incredibly careful to maintain healthy, regular sleep cycles. I know if I stay awake too late, or oversleep in the morning, I am at risk of becoming 'unhinged'.

Sleep–wake cycles were once largely dependent on the earth's cyclic activity. We only had natural light, and we slept when it was dark. Now we can have bedrooms lit up like a supernova, and can comfortably read, watch TV or any number of things until morning.

Circadian cycle regulation has been altered and this can be detrimental.

Circadian rhythm

So, what is circadian rhythm and why is it important? Circadian rhythm is an approximate 24-hour cycle in the physiological functioning and biological processes (physical, mental and behavioural changes) of humans, plants, animals and cyanobacteria. It's sometimes called our internal clock. The rhythm can be modulated by sunlight and season, and is integral in determining our sleep and eating patterns.

But due to artificial lighting, time-zone travel, shift work and socialising, our circadian rhythm can be well and truly messed up. Disturbances to circadian rhythms are associated with a greater risk of mood disorders (such as depression and bipolar disorder), reduced or worse subjective feelings of wellbeing, and slower reaction times.[228]

Knowing whether we are a night owl or a morning lark is important in establishing the right lifestyle factors to best support a healthy mind. It's also important to adopt consistent sleep patterns — and this includes weekends. The discrepancy between sleep habits kept during the week and those on the weekend is referred to as social jetlag. Misalignment of the circadian rhythm due to social jetlag does *not* encourage mental health and wellbeing.[229]

Another misalignment for human biology and the modern world is exposure to blue light, which emits from our smartphones, laptops and tablet screens. An overload of blue light will interrupt the production of melatonin (an important hormone that tells our body when it's time to sleep).[230]

Tricking the chickens

We bought chickens in winter, before they had started laying. Weeks went by and still no eggs, and we were left wondering if our new additions, although lovely, were duds. My husband read that a strategy to promote egg laying in winter (chickens may go off the lay in the cold months, or in our case delay the commencement of egg laying) was to set up lights in the chicken coop to go on at sunset, so that the chickens would be tricked into thinking that the days were longer and that winter was over. And it worked ... we tricked the chickens with light. Every morning there were eggs in the nesting boxes, even on the coldest wintery days.

Unfortunately, just like the ease with which we tricked our chickens, blue light tricks our brain that it's day, therefore we wake right up when we shouldn't.

There is a way to minimise the effects of blue light before sleep. Researchers at the University of Toronto compared the melatonin levels of people exposed to bright indoor light who were wearing blue-light–blocking glasses, to people exposed to regular dim light without wearing glasses. Levels of melatonin were about the same in the two groups, which strengthens the hypothesis that blue light is a suppressor of melatonin, and indicates that investing in some blue-light-blocking glasses is worthwhile.[231]

Although they say that seven to nine hours of sleep is most favourable for health, most research indicates the quality of sleep that you get is more important.[232]

~

Tips for good quality sleep

- Do not consume caffeine after 3 p.m.

- Protect yourself from blue light by wearing blue-light blocking glasses in the evening.

- Don't use electronic devices two to three hours before bed, keep electronic devices out of your bedroom, and use blackout curtains.

- Use supplements such as magnesium. Supplementing with magnesium can enhance the quality of sleep. It does this by reducing stress and may help regulate melatonin. I use 800 milligrams of magnesium a day.

- If you do sleep with a phone in your room, turn it on airplane mode.

- Another great supplement is GABA (see page 145), which functions as a neurotransmitter in the brain and has a calming effect, which is great for sleep.

Movement

Exercise is a celebration of what our body can do, and movement is a valuable tool in the arsenal for achieving mental wellness. In fact, there is a glut of evidence suggesting we need to engage in physical activity in order to be mentally well.[233]

Movement patterns have changed considerably in modern times, with exercise now being a scheduled activity rather than functional. Our early ancestors had to run, walk (for miles), crawl, lift, throw and climb on a daily basis to survive. We often sit in front of screens for long periods in artificial lighting, both during the day at work, and then in the evening for entertainment. For a healthy, well mind we need to spend quality time outdoors, walking, playing and moving.

I credit my high level of physical activity as saving me from a breakdown on many occasions. When I am moving my body I can calm my mind, and have found that it is therapeutic to move and sweat.

In my 30s I took up ultra-running, the definition of ultra being distances over a traditional marathon. Ultra-running took my need to move my body to a new place, as many ultra-events take place on trails out in the bush. The rhythmic pounding on undulating terrain gave my mind the meditative environment it needed to be still. I was hooked. I am not a fast runner and so was never at the front of the pack, but that didn't matter — I felt calm, centred and alive. There was no bipolar voice or mental chaos out on a trail and often, even after 100 kilometres of running outdoors, and with a tired and beaten-up body, I would be sad that my quiet time had ended.

Now, I am certainly not suggesting you take up ultra-running; it is actually quite pro-inflammatory and can create havoc for gut health. But I cannot stress enough the importance of physical activity for a well mind. Studies have reported that exercise is not only beneficial for those with mental illness, but that it is a great strategy for mental wellness, for most.[234]

Any type of movement can be beneficial, and getting outdoors is the most therapeutic setting. A study recently published in the *American Journal of Psychiatry* highlights that exercise, even just an hour a week, can deliver significant protection against depression. The study followed 33,309 adults for eleven years and concluded that if causality is assumed, and there are no other major cofounders, at least 12 percent of new cases of depression could be prevented if all adults participated in at least one hour of physical activity each week.[235] I would argue that one hour per week is not enough, and that we should use every opportunity available to move our body: regardless, this data is encouraging.

As with everything, moderation is key. Those for whom excessive physical activity can be harmful are those who suffer tendencies towards the extreme, such as addictive overtraining, or those with exaggerated preoccupation with physical appearance.[236] Other than those exceptions, exercise is beneficial for our mind, because not only does it pump blood to the brain, it also increases connections between the nerves in the brain and increases the size of the hippocampus, which helps to regulate the amygdala, and gives context for memories. When the hippocampus is functioning well it buffers stress both internally and from our environment.[237]

What is of vital importance, especially to those of us aiming for excellent mental health and emotional wellbeing, is that exercise reduces inflammation — chronic inflammation, the kind that is harmful to our mind. It has been reported in a study published in *Brain, Behaviour and Immunity* that just 20–30 minutes of brisk walking can significantly reduce inflammation.[238] We know that people who exercise regularly have fewer symptoms of depression and anxiety than those who don't, and that moderate-intensity exercise can be an effective treatment on its own for mental illness.[239]

~

Move for your mind

What is your favourite type of exercise? Swimming, walking, dancing, surfing, team sports? Conduct your own experiment. Next time you are feeling unwell in your mind, force yourself (it may be hard, but just do it as a test) to engage in some form of exercise. Keep it up for 30–40 minutes. Before you walk out the door, record how you feel inside your mind. When you get home go straight to the pen and paper and again record how you feel. I would make a bet that you feel at least 70 percent better than you did before you left.

CHAPTER 10:

Epigenetics

'Epigenetics doesn't change the genetic code, it changes how that's read. Perfectly normal genes can result in cancer or death. Vice-versa, in the right environment, mutant genes won't be expressed. Genes are equivalent to blueprints; epigenetics is the contractor. They change the assembly, the structure.'

Bruce Lipton

I have only just recently, in my 40s, met my two half-sisters (as mentioned, I never got to meet my biological father), and fortunately it has been an interesting and happy journey. We have had endless conversations about similarities between us — there are many — and also questions relating to potential genetic predisposition to illness that I may have inherited from my father. I now have insight into where some of my idiosyncrasies come from (some of which I had previously attributed to bipolar; it is nice to know they are not).

With regard to genetic predisposition to disease, I was nervous to ask the questions. What if he had suffered cancer, Alzheimer's or other devastating diseases? Will these be passed down? And it's not just the genes associated with disease that are important, but also genes associated with past trauma.[240]

And we used to believe that if we had the gene, we would get ill and have to take a pill. This is no longer the case, with new research indicating that good nutrition, adequate sleep, meditation, reducing alcohol intake and minimising exposure to environmental toxins can have a positive effect on our health, both physically and mentally.

Epigenetics is a new and exciting area of research that focuses on the mechanisms for how genes are switched on and off, without any changes in the DNA of the cell. We now know that this occurs when we make lifestyle changes. Dr Rudolph Tanzi, professor of neurology at Harvard University Medical School, wrote the book *Super Genes* with Dr Deepak Chopra, global leader in the field of mind–body medicine.

They write:

Only 5% of disease-related gene mutations are fully deterministic, while 95% can be influenced by diet, behavior, and other environmental conditions. Current models of wellbeing largely ignore genes, yet studies have shown that a program of positive lifestyle changes alter 4000 to 5000 different gene activities.[241]

As mentioned, we now know that epigenetic change can be passed down from parent to child through generations.[242] This means that if our parents or grandparents experienced trauma in their lives, we too may experience adverse health effects from that trauma.

The genetic changes due to generational trauma can be reversed with some work. There is evidence that enriching our environment leads to increased levels of glucocorticoid receptors (GR), so it's a good place to start.[243] But what does this mean in practical terms?

~

Trauma reversed via regulation of GR

When a body senses danger it releases a glucocorticoid, a hormone that adjusts heart rate, brain function and energy production during stress. Glucocorticoid binds to the glucocorticoid receptors (GR) in nerve cells of the brain. Normally the binding will shut off glucocorticoid production so that the stress response ceases.

However, the gene for the receptor is inactive in those who have experienced childhood stress. Without GR to bind to, the hormone continues to be released and the stress continues, after the threat has subsided.[244]

A place to heal

So, what exactly is an enriched environment where we can heal our mind? Most studies have been in rodent models, and have involved strategies such as increasing novel food, providing bigger cages, exercise wheels, or increasing group size for greater sociability.[245] Other studies in humans have included mindfulness meditation,[246] music lessons[247] or physical activity.[248] These studies have shown that the enrichment promotes improved endocrine, neuronal and behavioural functions. In other words, where there is generational trauma manifesting as chronic stress, poor health of our mind is likely to follow. But we *can* heal. For example, if childhood stress occurs, it may track through life and result in endocrine dysfunction in adulthood, which leads to a number of adverse health effects. By incorporating strategies to enrich our environment, we can reverse the adverse effects.

Can you remember a time you felt really low and have been dragged (or managed to drag yourself) outdoors? Perhaps to the beach or for a walk in a park? Slowly, little by little, depression, panic or anxiety just melt away and you are transformed. You can see the beauty everywhere: really see it. You sink into a meditative state, and your brainwaves change.

Researchers looking at the central nervous system and the way that time in nature influences our fight-or-flight response have reported encouraging results. In these studies stress hormones, respiration, heart rate and sweating measurements suggest that short doses of nature can calm our farm[249] (Aussie slang for stress less).

In fact, a recent study in the United Kingdom, involving 95,000 participants across ten cities, reported a protective effect on depression from hanging out in greenery, showing that those living in leafier communities are 4 percent less likely to suffer from a major depressive disorder.[250] That is significant when most of us have access to some parkland.

Japan has made *shinrin-yoku* — 'forest bathing'— a part of its national public health program since 1982. Forest bathing means walking and spending time in nature (it sounds like heaven). Forest bathing helps us reconnect and become grounded. Over the course of eight years, Japanese officials studied the physiological and psychological impact of forest bathing. When compared to hanging out in the city, they found that levels of the stress hormone, cortisol, dropped after participants spent just 30 minutes immersed in nature.[251]

I have experienced these amazing effects first-hand, and believe that the time I have invested getting out and running on forest trails or tree-lined streets has been essential in my journey towards a well mind. Just 30 minutes can be the difference between a negative, stress-filled mindset and a healthy, positive perspective.

'Silent' treatments

I have a Christian faith, love Buddhist principles and do intrinsically believe in a higher being who loves us and wants to be one with us. I recall that during my younger years when I had a regular silent practice I was calmer, and managed my mind better than when I neglected prayer and meditation. I have recently started to get up 30–40 minutes earlier than usual so I can spend time alone in the stillness of dawn. And I have to say, that the improvement in the wellbeing of my mind has been phenomenal.

Sitting with my mind has been confronting, and all kinds of things come up: it's extraordinarily uncomfortable. But, through this practice I have gained insight into the things that trigger me emotionally and I feel like I can slow things down in my head.

A recent review published in *Frontiers in Immunology* has looked at the mechanisms by which different mind–body intervention (including yoga and meditation) influence gene expression.[252] The researchers conclude that a total of 18 studies demonstrate changes on a molecular level that benefit our mind and body, accompanying meditation. The review honed into changes in certain proteins accompanying gene activation during meditation, which can have significant effects on the brain and immune system.

We know that when we are stressed our fight-or-flight is triggered — think back to the cavemen fleeing that lion — we have an increase in the production of nuclear factor kappa B (NF-kB), and NF-kB regulates how our genes are expressed. This clever little molecule activates genes to produce inflammatory cytokines, which, if the stress only lasts a little while (until we outrun that tiger or lion, or whatever) is no big deal. But the problem is that we are under constant stress these days, and so this chronic inflammation leads to a host of issues such as poor mind and emotional health.

According to the review, those who engage in regular prayer, meditation or yoga have a decrease in production of NF-kB and inflammatory cytokines, which leads to a reversal of the highly inflammatory gene expression pattern, and reduces risk of inflammatory disease states.

Compelling results were also reported in an earlier study from the journal *Psychoneuroendocrinology*, where meditation significantly reduced inflammation,[253] and a 2012 study reported different patterns of DNA activation, possibly reflecting epigenetic changes, during periods of self-reported 'higher states of consciousness' compared to ordinary awareness.[254] Following are two meditation exercises that I do regularly. It took a while to build up this practice and I had to start with just five minutes because I couldn't settle my mind. I have now worked my way up to 40 minutes — so, be patient with yourself. I do this first thing in the morning, but you can do it any time.

~

Meditation exercise: Focusing the mind

Pour yourself a big glass of warm water with a squeeze of lemon juice. Find a comfy spot and sit with your back supported.

Now, breathe in for four counts and exhale for eight counts. Repeat this pattern and keep it going for 30 breaths. While you are focusing on your breathing, also hone in on your senses: what you are hearing and feeling at that time, in that moment. Focus on being in the present moment. Your thoughts will drift off, of course, and that is normal; thinking is something we do automatically.

Rather than attempting to cease thinking, focus on a word or thought such as 'love' or 'peace' or 'truth', and just use that word to catch your thoughts. You can say it out loud or just think it, and as your thoughts start to drift into, 'Why on earth am I up so early ... What is that noise? ... I wish I had sent that email to Joe last night ... Did I feed the cat? ... I'm cold, wish I had put my dressing gown on ... What is that noise ... Seriously, I suck at meditation ... Is time up yet?' you can gently drift back to the word of your choice and let your mind empty again. When the thoughts come in, observe them, and then let them drift out and go back to your chosen word.

~

Meditation exercise: Sweeping out the debris

I often feel that my mind is like a hoarder's house, with stuff everywhere. Too scared to be alone and quiet, I didn't want to face the disaster zone in my head: this exercise helps.

I begin with my breathing exercise and focus on my word being 'truth', and then when I feel in the 'zone' I imagine my mind (for me it looks like a dome-shaped space). With an image of my messy, untidy, disorganized, hectic mind, I arm myself with a huge broom. I go into the huge dome-shaped space and switch on some lights, and sweep everything away. I don't sort through the mess, I just sweep, and it all gets swept over a big cliff that I don't look at. It doesn't take long (cleaning my mind isn't in real time), and then I am left with an immense (looks so much bigger empty), dome-shaped space that is now incandescent.

I then take my time and put a few things in the corner of the big empty space. I put my dreams there. I place love there, and repeat that I am loved and I give love. I place the image of what I want to give to the world. I place my financial dreams, my spiritual dreams, my career dreams, all in the corner of this big white space, and then I look at it all and give thanks.

Yes, it may sound a bit out there, but these strategies have science behind them and have helped me significantly. It is difficult to take that first step, but once you do, you will continue to move ahead.

(You may take one step forward, two back, but keep trying, you *will* get there!) I never thought I would be able to meditate, and it's called a practice for a reason. But now I can't imagine not investing the time for my mind.

Another fundamental aspect of enriching our environment is taking stock of the people we hang out with.

The people we mix with

I have lost friends throughout my life. Some by choice, others because I just wasn't very nice to be around. I believe that people come into our lives for a season and we can impart something to them, and learn something from them.

We usually gravitate towards those who make us feel good, or those with similar interests. However, sometimes we find ourselves in constant communion with those who drain our energy and our passion for life. A popular saying (supported by evidence) is 'We become who we spend the most time with.'[255] We are more likely to grow negative when we are exposed to negative chatter daily, and cynical if we are enveloped in cynicism. Conversely, being in contact with emotionally healthy people can rub off and have a positive impact.

The idea of making healthy choices about who we spend time with can create some ethical dilemmas. For example: you have been friends with Samantha since you were nineteen, having been through thick and thin, experiencing breakups and heartache, weddings and funerals. Sam has always been part of your life. You were living in separate cities after Sam got married and moved away, but you remained in regular contact. You are both now in your 40s and Sam's husband just got a transfer back to your home city. You are so excited, as even though you pick up on the fact that you and Sam no longer share key values, and are complete opposites on many levels, she is your bestie and now you will be able to hang out all the time.

The bad news is that after spending more time with Sam you feel emotionally drained. Samantha is not emotionally healthy and has no desire to improve her mental wellbeing. She appears to be floating in a victim mentality, and has no interest in nourishing her body or her mind. In fact, she appears to be hellbent on pulling you down and is endlessly criticising you. You don't feel good after spending time with her, but she is your oldest friend and you can't just ditch her, can you?

I would argue that you can. Oprah once said, 'Surround yourself with only people who are going to lift you higher.'[256] Spending so much time with Sam detrimentally affects the wellbeing of your mind. Would you spend time with someone who was making you physically sick? The people we spend time with collectively make up our environment, and as such, to enrich our environment means that we need to choose wisely who we hang out with.

The famous Roman politician and philosopher Cicero gave us a compelling guide to finding, and appreciating, friends.[257] Cicero points out that we can't thrive when isolated, because we will stagnate and become unable to see ourselves as we are. So, we do need to have contact with others. He proposes that a true friend will challenge us to become better, because they appreciate the potential inside us. I like this — I believe it is crucial to surround ourselves with those who encourage us to grow and be the best that we can be.

The Principle of Progressive Resistance — used in exercise science — refers to the body's ability to adapt and respond to the demands placed on it. The principle is based on the premise that the muscles need to be challenged to grow, and they will progressively improve to overcome any increasing resistance. We can extrapolate this to our minds as well. We need to be challenged intellectually, spiritually and relationally, and if we are in contact with individuals who challenge us on these levels, we will progressively grow and strengthen our mind.

While it is common advice to surround ourselves with people who think similarly to us, exclusively including like-minded people in your inner circle isn't a great idea. Imagine how boring and uninspiring life would be if our friends all had exactly the same likes, dislikes, goals and dreams? Instead we should focus on 'like' values, such as integrity, honesty and commitment. And as Cicero advises, surrounding ourselves with people who inspire us and challenge us, and make us accountable, is crucial for mental and emotional wellbeing.

The next section is the icing on the cake.

We have covered tools that will form the foundation for transforming our mindset and changing our reality — our food, gut health, stress levels, sleep, exercise and more. Now we can work on altering our perspective.

Changing our mindset is the key to moving through tough life situations with gratitude and peace.

PART 3:
TOOLS TO ENRICH

CHAPTER 11:

Meaning and Purpose

'We moderns have an arsenal of tranquillisers and painkillers at our disposal, but our expectations of ease and pleasure, and our intolerance of inconvenience and discomfort, have increased to such an extent that we may well suffer from pain more than our ancestors ever did.'

Yuval Noah Harari

In the depths of darkness I have battled to find meaning and purpose. Exploring the meaning of life and one's purpose can seriously send one crazy. I've felt like an empty shell often, but I can recall a time where I had a bit of an epiphany. If I was empty, then I could be filled with anything. I was a blank canvas and could paint my purpose from scratch.

We create our purpose. Being alive affords us opportunity to find out what is important to us, but often we have to suffer during the process.

The idea of humans finding meaning through suffering was exemplified by Viktor E Frankl (1905–1997).[258] Frankl was a Jewish psychiatrist who in 1942 was sent to Theresienstadt concentration camp with his family. He was later separated from his wife, stripped of all he had, and sent to the Nazi concentration camp at Auschwitz. After surviving the horror of the Holocaust, and witnessing the unyielding strength of the human spirit, he wrote one of the most important books ever written, *Man's Search for Meaning* (1946). The reason this book is so remarkable is because it gives us insight into human nature when faced with the unthinkable.

Frankl kept his psychiatry hat on through the horrific ordeal in Auschwitz, and noted that the prisoners who fixated on their past found no reason to hope; they saw their spiritual selves dissolve in the horror they were experiencing. Therefore, they couldn't see beyond their harrowing circumstances to a future. Those prisoners adopted the belief that life was over, and that any opportunity for growth and meaningful existence was no longer possible in the present. Though a seemingly impossible task, Frankl concluded that the prisoners who *embraced* the devastating challenges encountered daily, and still grasped at meaning in each present day, were better off than those who clung to their past life and wasted away.

Frankl, a strong proponent of Nietzsche's philosophy 'He who has a why to live for can bear with almost any how,' argues that a sense of purpose or meaning can get you through anything. Frankl also writes, *'They offer sufficient proof that everything can be taken from a man but one thing: the last of the human freedoms — to choose one's attitude in any given set of circumstances, to choose one's own way.'*[259]

We have no control over people or the circumstances that we encounter daily, but we do have the freedom to choose how we respond.

~

Of course we have all heard of Abraham Lincoln, the 16th President of the United States. He led the country through the Civil War and paved the way for the abolition of slavery.

You may not know that Lincoln suffered debilitating depression. Robert L Wilson,[260] who served in the Illinois legislature with Abraham Lincoln, shed some light on the health and wellbeing of the 16th President's mind and stated that he was overcome with mental depression.[261] Who would have thought!

Modern clinicians, using the standard diagnostic criteria, agree that Lincoln suffered with depression. But how did Lincoln wrestle with the monsters in his head?

Lincoln didn't hide his depression, but he did have strategies in place to help overcome his unwell mind. He used humour and storytelling, and confided in others when he was really struggling. Lincoln learned to live with his depressive disposition well before Prozac was invented. Lincoln wrote to Quintin Campbell, the son of his wife's cousin, who was feeling dissatisfied with life, 'Adhere to your purpose, and you will soon feel as well as you ever did.'[262]

We can learn from Abraham Lincoln that a crucial ingredient for a well mind is a sense of purpose and meaning.

I have always been fascinated by great thinkers throughout history. One of my favourites is Aristotle, who coined the phrase 'eudaimonia' for his idea of happiness. However, rather than just the pursuit of feeling good all the time, Aristotle's idea of eudaimonia is reflected in the pursuit of virtue, excellence and the best within us, and it's an idea that has weathered the test of time.

Psychologist Alan Waterman and colleagues came up with the concept of eudaimonic wellbeing (EWB), and developed a eudaimonic wellbeing scale (QEWB).[263] The QEWB measures: our sense of meaning and purpose in life — which describes the personally meaningful objectives that we direct our talents and skills toward; enjoyment derived from activities that are 'personally expressive'; intense involvement in activities — not just any activities or hobbies, but those that are related to our life goals; perceived development of own best potentials (virtuous potential); and investment of significant effort towards achieving excellence.

To achieve the sense of meaning and wellbeing that Aristotle describes we must follow a manner of living and pursuits that promote wellness and vitality, and allow us to thrive. Below is a worksheet to help you identify the personally meaningful factors in your life, and how you can develop these areas.

Meaning and purpose

Choose 'very important', 'neutral' or 'not important' for each category	very important	neutral	not important
Family			
Career			
Recreation			
Health and wellness			
Personal growth			
Helping others			
Socialising			

Next to each factor write 'very important', 'neutral' or 'not important'. For the factors you have labelled 'very important', I want you to do a little self-reflection, and expand.

For example, I rate health and wellness as very important, so I will reflect on why I find value in that. I find value because to be fit and healthy gives me the means to be the best that I can be and assists me in keeping my mind well. And if I feel the best that I can, then I will be more present for others in my life. I will feel good in myself, and that positively impacts my mood, and so then I am likely to help others feel good.

When you have identified very important and important factors, and reflected on why you find value in them, think about the amount of time you devote to each. For example, if you rate helping others as very important, and the reason is that you like to see others happy, do you manage to find time to do this, and is the time spent adequate? If the answer is no, consider the time spent on factors you rate as neutral or not important. Could time be transferred from less important factors to factors that will impart a sense of meaning for your life?

In the example of helping others, consider ways you might do this. Are there charity organisations you could join? Do you have an elderly neighbour you could offer to run errands for? Some life adjustment may be necessary to allow the transfer of your time, but in shifting focus to factors that you rate as important, or very important in your life, you allow purpose and meaning to enter into your day.

Happiness accompanies a sense of purpose and meaning, but sometimes this involves an element of suffering. Work out what you are willing to suffer for. My example of health and wellness comes at a price. I get up early every morning to meditate/pray and then exercise, because these practices help me to be healthy in my mind and body. I don't just eat everything I crave, because I understand that my health will suffer — but sometimes I would love to eat pizza for breakfast. Nothing worth having comes easily, but when we can find meaning and value in what we are doing, life is a little rosier.

Meaning in the everyday

I once heard a story about a doctor who was reminiscing on his days as an intern in a large hospital. While he was finishing up after the night shift, a cleaner would arrive to clean the surgical theatre. The then young intern noticed that the cleaner was always cheery; the doctor could feel happiness radiating from him. He often mused that the cleaner (who, let's face it, didn't have the best job) appeared far happier than any of his colleagues who were surgeons at this well-known hospital.

One early morning, the intern had a chance to chat to the cleaner and said, 'Hey man, you always seem so happy — what's the secret?' The cleaner just laughed and said, 'Well, notice how clean this operating theatre is after I have finished? You surgeons need lots of light to see what you're doing when saving all the lives that you save. And notice how the light reflects off the clean floor? Because I do my job so well, you surgeons can do your job well, and save so many lives. And I don't have half the stress that you do.' It's all about perspective. The cleaner had found purpose and meaning in his work, and consequently found happiness.

I met my husband three years ago and moved in with him six weeks later (yes — impulsive). He has two children, and I became the primary caregiver. This is after successfully raising my own children into amazing humans, which any parent can attest takes some sacrifice and work. I had forgotten that bedtime takes such a long time … and hello, who is handing out the Valium at meal time? Don't even get me started on school lunches! Anyway, I gave up my career in academia (more on this shortly), and started to work from home so that my husband could work and we could give the kids some stability (one child is diagnosed with high-functioning autism and is prone to anxiety, so stability is important).

Now, it has taken three years to accept that my freedom has absconded, along with my spare time. I made the choices so didn't expect sympathy (not true — I felt like I should have been treated like Mother Teresa and worshipped like Queen Nefertiti), but I struggled — boy have I struggled.

The answer to my struggle has been to change my perspective and find meaning in my new role. My expertise is nutrition. Because I have knowledge of the powerful way food influences our mind and body, I can ensure that my stepchildren get the best possible nutrition to nourish their young minds. I can also give them stability and support. I am an open person, and I hope they will feel comfortable talking to me as a friend when they reach adolescence and adulthood. I have taken some of the load from my husband, and so I am enabling him to be less stressed and anxious, thus supporting his emotional health and wellness.

Focusing on these factors gives me a sense of purpose and meaning, rather than focusing on my 'lack' … My lack of freedom, alone time, career, et cetera. Again, this way of thinking is a practice: it doesn't come easily.

~

A question

What little thing can you pick out of your work or life that you see helps others? Think back to the story about the man who cleans the hospital. What part of your life can you view differently, and see that you make a greater contribution than you originally thought?

Purpose in the mundane

I spent much of my adult life believing that things I accomplish in life would give me a sense of purpose. After a tumultuous youth and dropping out of school at age fifteen, I was as proud as punch when I was awarded my PhD. I felt like I had overcome and that my achievements defined who I was. I got an ongoing appointment at a university in my home city, and was developing a nutrition course. This became my identity, and my ego was chuffed to bits.

Then, as mentioned, I quit and became a stay-at-home substitute parent, writing books in my pyjamas. Depression crept in slowly, something I am unaccustomed to — historically, the bipolar mania and depression are fast-moving little gremlins. It became harder to get up early, routine and schedules were lost, and I was really low. I felt such grief over a perceived loss of my identity.

Fortunately, because I had already done some internal work I could see that although my pain and grieving were valid, I was still the same person who had worked hard to overcome. But, I had to get back on track and find meaning and purpose in my new role.

There was also great risk involved. I love writing, but I am terrified of rejection: all writers deal with rejection! I get bored easily and am prone to isolation depression, so days at home in my pyjamas can be a problem. And I don't have a maternal bone in my body. To clarify, I have lots of love for my kids and stepkids, but zero interest in wiping snotty noses, cleaning up projectile vomit after a bout of gastro, attending parent–teacher interviews or sitting through school assemblies.

Mark Manson (I mentioned him earlier) writes a fantastic blog (if you don't mind some profanity). He wrote a post on seven strange questions to find your life purpose, suggesting that in the quest to find purpose we should ask ourselves: 'What's your favourite flavour of sh#t sandwich, and does it come with an olive?' What he means is, we have to accept that we are going to have downright lousy days regardless of what we do. There is always, *always* a poop sandwich. So, work out what kind of 'poop' you can endure while pursuing your passion — because there will plenty of it.

And it appears I can endure mundane domesticity and isolation, if it means I get to write.

In the same post Manson asks: 'If you knew you were going to die one year from today, what would you do and how would you want to be remembered?'

The topic of death is something we rarely want to explore, even in the context of living a life filled with meaning. One thing that has affected my decisions over the past couple of years, and propelled me on the path I have chosen, is the death of my former sister-in-law.

Michelle (or Pip as she was affectionately known) was diagnosed with an inoperable (and fast-growing) brain tumour. During those months after hearing of her illness, I started to question what was important in my own life. I realized that at the end of my life, I did not want to be remembered for how many research papers I had published, or how far up the ladder I had managed to crawl (and a crawl it would have been). I want to spend time with people I love and feel purpose in all that I do. We have one life and so we need to prioritize what is really important, or we will end up full of regret. It really is that simple.

Another hurdle that contributes to an unhealthy mind in so many ways is our habit of taking life too seriously. We ruminate and obsess over things that we may not even remember in months, or even weeks, let alone at the end of our time on earth. Do you think that while on your deathbed you will be thinking back to making that mistake at work, or the time someone criticized your decision, or when you didn't get a promotion you were so sure you deserved?

Reflect on this and ask yourself: 'Is this even going to matter in two weeks?' Taking the time to reflect will draw things into perspective.

CHAPTER 12:

Beyond Rumination

'The combination of rumination and negative thinking is toxic. Research shows that people who ruminate while sad or distraught are likely to feel besieged, powerless, self-critical, pessimistic, and generally negatively biased.'

Sonja Lyubomirsky

It may not surprise you to learn that I am a ruminator. In fact, I'm an awesome ruminator — if there was an award for ruminating, I would win it. It's one of the most boring things about me. I can take a negative thought or circumstance and unpack it every which way, over and over and over again. Boring as bat poop.

Rumination can be crudely defined as ongoing, cyclic and depressive thinking. It is the opposite of mental wellness. It is often the response to negative moods and is increasingly common.

'Why am I so moody? ... Why can't I cope with heartbreak? ... Why am I so slow? ... Why can't I cope with life?' is frequent dialogue in rumination. Some of us believe that if we ruminate we are essentially gaining insight into why we feel so bad. Or, we believe that rumination may help us prevent future mistakes.

Dr Costas Papageorgiou, a Chartered Clinical Psychologist of the British Psychological Society, as well as Chartered Scientist of the Science Council, and Dr Adrian Wells, Professor of Clinical and Experimental Psychopathology at the University of Manchester, came up with a model that proposed that positive beliefs about the advantages of rumination (for example, 'Ruminating helps me get insight into my depression.') are likely to result in the person jumping on the hamster wheel of rumination, and not being able to get off.[264] Once this occurs, the individual will then believe that the process is both uncontrollable and harmful ('It's impossible for me to not ruminate about the failures of the past.'), and likely to produce detrimental social consequences ('They don't like me because I ruminate so frequently.'). The activation of the negative beliefs then results in depression and anxiety.

Imagine you've had a great day at work, then fifteen minutes before you leave, your boss stops at your office door and asks if you finished the report he had asked you to write. You try to explain that you had to prioritize other things, and that you will have it to him by the end of the week. He shakes his head and firmly states that he needs it now, before storming off. You get on that hamster wheel and don't get off until you finally fall asleep at 2 a.m. You wake up the next day, remember with a feeling of dread, and then the rumination begins again: 'I'm going to lose my job ... I am so incompetent ... They can all see that I can't cope ... Why am I so stupid?'

And it's addictive (as well as boring). We need to stop, because it's a fatal factor for mental wellness. Before we can overcome ruminative thought patterns, we need some practice. When we become aware that we are in a ruminative rut, we should take some time to become fully aware of the thoughts as they run through our mind. A Thought Cloud meditation is a useful exercise, because it brings awareness to the thought.

~

Thought cloud meditation exercise

Take ten long slow breaths in and out.

On the last breath move your attention to your mind. What thoughts are travelling through? Are you excited, nervous, worried, confused, scared?

Let the thoughts just float around in your mind, much like a cloud. Decide what you want to do with that thought. Is it a thought you want to change, or do you just want to let it go? Think of the thought as a big cloud. It can float out of your head just as easily as it floated in.

You are in control of your thoughts, so if you don't want the thought there, let it float away.

It's important to acknowledge that rumination serves no purpose other than to damage the health of our mind, and with practice we can regain control of our thoughts and allow our mind some peace.

∼

Other ways to stop the habit of rumination

Question your thoughts. Will this affect you in the future? Is ruminating on the apparent problem going to solve it? What action can you take, rather than just repetitive thinking?

Think about the fact that the mind-damaging thought may not even be accurate.

Go for a walk, or hit the gym.

Rather than just letting the thought eat away at you, write down a plan of action. Be specific about how you can address the problem.

Then, take that action.

> Be kind to yourself. Talk to yourself as you would a friend.
>
> Think about the fact that you don't ruminate on good things, so why would you devote so much precious energy on the bad?
>
> Journal the thoughts out of your head and onto paper.

You also may have realized from reading thus far that I have been guilty of being explosive throughout my life. There were times I felt like I would disintegrate if I didn't let my emotional fire out of me. But that kind of reactivity is not beneficial, and after the anger has subsided I always wind up feeling oodles of regret. As mentioned, thoughts fuel our emotions and the thoughts are often a result of the stories programmed into our young minds early in life.

All it takes is a pause, a breath and some self-reflection to prevent an explosion, and instead have fruitful communication.

~

A pause before reaction

I have adopted this exercise to pause and think through the story I am reciting in my mind before I react to someone.

Next time you are in an argument with a partner, friend or family member, experiment with this.

You feel the emotion bubbling to the surface as something that has been said triggers you. Now, stop. Breathe in for four counts and out for eight counts. Think. Get curious. What is it that they said that upset you? What story has it drawn out for you? What emotions are you feeling?

Keep breathing, and feel those feelings. Name them. If it's anger, ask yourself where the anger comes from. Does it come from fear? Jealousy? Shame? Sadness? Vulnerability?

What story is playing in your mind? For example, 'He thinks I'm stupid and is trying to make me feel dumb.' 'They don't like me.' 'They never listen to what I'm saying.' Take time to understand that you are attaching a feeling to the event.

Then, start your response with, 'The story playing in my mind is that you think I am ... This makes me feel ...'

Now, ask the person in question to explain their behaviour so you can understand their perspective.

This response feels so much better than the stress associated with a full-on fight and will likely resolve the situation much more quickly.

CHAPTER 13:

Don't Fight It — Just Feel It

'In this book, not only is there no happy ending, there is no happy beginning and very few happy things in the middle.'

Lemony Snicket [265]

Universal law — where there is good, there is also bad. And vice versa. So, we can't avoid struggle or pain, and we are never going to feel happy all the time. We just need accept it, which takes practice. A crucial skill for a healthy mind is to learn to live with our emotional turmoil, and learn to accept the full range of human experience. The alternative is to simply experience that with which we cannot deal.

To suffer elevates us to a degree that we would not attain if we were to be comfortable and happy all through life. Suffering offers growth. In fact, Russell Razzaque argues in his book *Breaking Down is Waking Up*[266] that experiencing a breakdown, or emotional/mental illness can be incredibly transformative, reminiscent of William James's twice born 'sick souls'.

American mindfulness teacher and neuroscience research consultant Shinzen Young states that 'suffering equals pain times resistance'.[267] The more we resist, the more we suffer. Of course we are going to resist to an extent, because we are human and we don't want to suffer — but we have to resign ourselves to the fact that at times life is going to suck.

We should endeavour to allow the negative thoughts to exist and acknowledge them. To walk through the negative, sad or painful experience builds strength and resilience. To get curious and reflect on why we feel those emotions is mind changing. 'Curiosity' is key here, because it motivates us to question.

~

Shift to curiosity

When you experience a negative emotion, take some time out.

Find a comfortable spot and sit with your eyes closed.

Take ten long, slow breaths. Look at the emotion you are feeling. Sit with it. Ask yourself: Why it is there? Is the emotion worth taking action on? Is the emotion hurting you or affecting your quality of life? Will the uncomfortable emotion be present long enough to be important? Do you want the emotion to leave?

Really look at what you are feeling and where the feeling comes from. If you feel hurt after something was said, were the words spoken hurtful, or was it the feeling those words triggered, that hurt?

Emotions are like beach balls in water; we can push them down and push them down and push them down, but they will always resurface. We partake of this pointless exercise because we're told as kids it's wrong to express anger, rage, sadness, frustration or the like. So, we push it all down, until it all pops back up again. In many cases, our emotions serve to protect us. Our anger can alert others to back off and leave us be. Our sadness can alert us to the fact that something is amiss and action needs to be taken to right a situation. Ignoring what we feel doesn't make it go away: the feelings will manifest in other ways, such as symptoms of anxiety, apathy and depression.

We need to get to a place where we can question the feelings as they come up, work out what the feelings are, where they came from, whether they are important, and actually give them a name.

When we name an emotion it gives us the space to have perspective, and is a powerful way to regain control. Rather than avoiding or resisting the emotion, we can name the resistance and then choose how to respond to the emotion.

According to UCLA Professor of Psychology Mathew Leiberman, when we name something we move blood flow to the prefrontal cortex (the centre of our brain for emotion regulation and perspective), away from the amygdala, which is where the reactions to emotions are born (see page 71). A study conducted by Leiberman and colleagues showed that labelling feelings can significantly diminish emotional reactivity arising from the amygdala.[268]

Psychologist and author Joan Rosenberg, in her book *90 Seconds to a Life You Love*, proposes that the eight common negative[269] feelings are: sadness, shame, helplessness, vulnerability, anger, embarrassment, disappointment and frustration.[270] These are common spontaneous reactions to things that don't occur the way we want, or expect. They rise up repeatedly, so we push them back down, because we don't want to experience the physical effects of the emotion. The feelings are uncomfortable, so we try hard to avoid them. But the problem is that the feelings affect our thoughts, just as our thoughts cause our feelings, and therefore this produces a constant loop. If we can just ride the 90-second wave of discomfort that the feelings produce, we can overcome the cycle that causes us to re-loop the feeling over and over again.

Rosenberg also talks about 'soulful disconnect'. This is the outcome of pushing down our feelings, thus disconnecting from them. Once we disconnect from the feelings — our feelings — we disengage from ourselves. If we are disconnected from ourselves, how on earth can we have healthy connections with anyone? Feeling disconnected leads to an unwell mind.

Let's make peace with the negative thoughts, rather than run from them.

If our primary focus is being happy and positive all the time, we aren't learning the skills to live in the world as it is. Life's beauty and fragility are intertwined; we need the skills to cope with the good and the bad.

CHAPTER 14:

Serving Others

'Helping others is the way we help ourselves.'

Oprah Winfrey

That's right, if you want a well mind, develop an altruistic mindset. This is an age-old principle encompassed in all major religions. Buddha instructed, 'Go your ways, oh monks, for the benefit of many, for the happiness of many, out of compassion for the world, for the good, benefit and happiness of gods and men.'

And the Bible, James 1:27, pronounces: 'Religion that is pure and undefiled before God, the Father, is this: to visit orphans and widows in their affliction, and to keep oneself unstained from the world.'

Regardless of your creed, the message is clear in instruction: help others. And it works. Living selfishly leads to dissatisfaction and disconnection, which eventually leads to pain. Conversely, focusing on others leads to connection and inner joy, and creates meaning in our life.

As you practise being of service, good things start to happen quite quickly. And mentally we flourish.

A 2003 study reported that 200 hours a year of volunteering to help others reduces the risk of hypertension and increases psychological wellbeing.[271] There is also a systematic review indicating that volunteer work can reduce depression, and improve life satisfaction and wellbeing.[272] Popular culture drives forth the message that looking after number one first will increase our happiness. What if it works the other way around?

Two recent studies have demonstrated that spending money on others will have a greater impact on wellbeing than spending money on oneself.[273] Another study highlights that acts of kindness in the workplace reduce depression in the givers, and increase life satisfaction — as well as prompting the receivers to pay the kindness forward.[274]

It may be that performing acts of kindness works as a 'well mind' tool because it impacts our self-perception and encourages us to view ourselves as kind and capable. Helping others may help us to realize our strengths and identify talents that we hadn't previously been aware of. And of course seeing others benefit from our service is priceless. It expands our world significantly and can only benefit our mental wellbeing.

As we serve others, we grasp the understanding that the world works in our favour and the rewards are self-fulfilling. Focusing solely on ourselves simply leads to discomfort and dissatisfaction with life and makes our world very small, which magnifies small problems that keep us low. To expand our world and our mind we need to get out there and find someone to help as a regular practice.

~

Some ways to be of service

Be present with others and listen. There is so much power in being present, because it makes someone in need feel validated and understood. In these busy times it's so easy to fly through conversations, which results in meaningless and superficial banter. Rather, let others know that you have time for them by being truly present in your conversations.

Volunteer your services. You may not want to help out at soup kitchens or volunteer in an aged care facility, and that's fine. There are many other ways of helping others. For example, if you are good with technology and consider yourself creative, you could offer your services to set up a website for a non-profit organization.

Be a mentor. Part of this role requires you to inspire and uplift someone. To challenge others and lift them out of their comfort zone is sometimes one of the best things you can do for someone.

Keep an eye out on little things that may make someone's day brighter. If you live close to your neighbours, take out their bin as well as your own. Drop in on an elderly neighbour. Offer to water someone's plants when they go away. Give a compliment to a stranger. Offer to give your time to someone for a whole day and let them plan what they would like to do. There is an abundance of little things we can do to help out others.

Donate a blog post.

Cook a meal for a friend.

Connect two friends or work colleagues who you know would get along.

The list is endless.

CHAPTER 15:

Gratefulness is
Mind Medicine

'The struggle ends when gratitude begins.'

Neale Donald Walsch

Gratitude is magic, and if we all practised gratitude the world would be different. You have probably heard this many times, and that's because it works. Much of the time, it's about perspective. For example, an income of US$32,400 per year would place you among the top 1 percent of income earners in the world.[275] Disease, poverty, famine and war claim thousands of lives, and yet here we are alive, with food on our plate and clean drinking water. There are so many things to be grateful for, and research supports the theory that gratitude will encourage a well mind,[276] and those who practise gratitude report greater wellbeing and have a more positive mood.[277]

A recent study involved participants writing a few sentences each week, focusing on specific topics. One group wrote about things they were grateful for that had occurred during the week. A second group wrote about daily irritations or things that had upset them. And a third group wrote about the events that had affected them (control group). After ten weeks, those who listed what they were grateful for were more optimistic and felt better about their lives. And, they also exercised more frequently, and had fewer visits to the doctor than those who focused on sources of irritation.[278] There are many such studies that show that simply being thankful for the small things can have huge positive effects on the wellbeing of our mind.[279]

Every morning I ask my stepchildren to tell me two things they are grateful for, and I do the same. Some mornings we get a bit stuck, but that is usually because we are trying not to be repetitive, or we want to come up with a doozy (the ego is always there — even in gratitude).

There is also evidence that taking another approach — mental subtraction — works wonders.[280] Mental subtraction is when you imagine what life would be like if the positive event hadn't happened. For example, you are grateful that you work close to where you live so that you don't have a tedious commute daily. Imagine if that wasn't the case and you worked 90 minutes from home. Mental subtraction helps us to bathe in gratitude as we imagine how difficult life could be without the comforts that we have.

Gratitude, like everything, is something to practise and grow. And it will change your mind.

~

Gratitude practices

Keep a gratitude journal and each week try to write five things for which you are grateful. Be specific and include why you are grateful.

Write thank-you notes to those who have had a positive impact on your life.

Identify three things you are grateful for about yourself. It may be as simple as, 'I'm so grateful that my legs get me from place to place,' or 'I'm grateful that I can remember important events.'

Imagine if something you value in your life suddenly disappeared. Now be grateful that it's still there.

Wake up each day and give thanks that you are living and breathing.

Gratitude is a good place to finish. We live in very privileged times in Western culture, yet we lose sight as we are caught up in fear and worry.

We have more control than we believe, but in most cases we give control away. We give it away to doctors, to food manufacturers, to social media and to buffers such as alcohol and junk food. If we can learn to be grateful even when things aren't going great, we will be on the way to possessing a well mind.

This all takes work, yes. But it's worth the investment. We don't have to travel through our precious lives feeling fear, shame, worry, anxiety, depression and discontent. I hope that my experiences and those I have passed on from others give you reason to believe that you can have a mind that is well.

CHAPTER 16:

We *Do* Have Control

*'It's your road, and yours alone. Others may walk
it with you, but no one can walk it for you.'*

Rumi

I was very mentally unwell. My days were filled with anxiety, anger,
fear, depression, self-doubt and self-loathing. I had a constant soul
ache and although I felt a desperate need for control over people
and things in my life, I felt I had no control over my inner turmoil.

Then one day it all changed. I didn't just wake and feel great; far
from it. I have had many relapses — embarrassing ones at that. There
was no standout epiphany pushing me to change. I simply reached
the point where I was sick of feeling low, sick of the tears, sick of

thinking 'What if?', and so sick of feeling like I could fragmentize at any time.

All it took was a decision.

The change didn't happen overnight. I had to work really hard. Nutrition, supplements, exercise, spiritual growth, removal of toxic people from my life, connection with others, positive self-talk and other healing modalities.

The more I have healed mentally, the more I have become aware of my potential.

All it took was that decision to start.

There have been many times I couldn't find hope in the world, but it wasn't because hope wasn't there; it was because my inner dialogue, my thoughts, the way I approached the world were blocking the light that shines brightly around hope. The work that I put into my body to maintain its health hadn't extended to my mind.

I have come across many people in recent years who are struggling with negativity, erratic moods, anxiety and depression. Most of us trudge through life and never question if we are feeling well in our mind, or if we could feel better.

We *can* feel better, and it *is* in our hands to do so. Our thoughts govern our feelings, and I want to emphasize that we are the only ones who have control over our thoughts; not our parents, our friends, our lovers, our kids.

It's often enticing to seek comfort over growth, but comfort doesn't last — growth does. The primitive part of our brain whines in the background of the chatter in our head with 'Don't-do-it-you'll-look-dumb-go-on-eat-the-junk-posing-as-food-bad-things-are-going-to-happen-so-don't-dare-relax-don't-say-how-you-really-feel-it's-too-dangerous-you-can't-do-that-there's-too-much-risk.' We have the power to override that primitive brain.

So, where do we go from here?

You have an arsenal of tools and an understanding that the health of your mind shapes your experience of this precious life. It's never too late to care for and nourish your mind. Start with being curious, and notice your thoughts. Notice the stories and recognize them for what they are, before they take hold. Use gratitude as medicine, use food as medicine and give your mind the reverence it deserves. Nourish with nutritious food, herbs and supplements. Care for the gut microbiome; it has much influence over what goes on in your head. Nourish with healthy thoughts, connect with nature and others, protect adequate time to sleep, exercise and develop a silent practice like breathwork or meditation.

And these are the ingredients to owning your mind and attaining mental wellness.

Appendix

Final Checklist

- No one is happier than anyone else. We are all getting by just how we can.

- We need to override the primitive wiring that motivates us to avoid discomfort and pain. When we face discomfort and pain head on, we experience life.

- Our feelings are caused by our thoughts, not by other people or circumstances. And we *can* control our thoughts.

- What we believe to be mental illness could just be a lack of mental wellness, and medication need not be the first point of call, unless in a state of crisis.

- We are wired to ruminate on the negative, and this is a built-in safeguard against putting ourselves in dangerous or uncomfortable situations.

- The stories we tell ourselves are not true.

- The food we eat affects the health and wellbeing of our mind.

Strategies

- Focus on three positive things that happen every day and discuss with family or friends.

- Believe that we can know ourselves, change ourselves and create new habits.

- Look for meaning and purpose even in the mundane.

- Be curious and reflect on negative emotions. Journal, talk and explore them.

- Practise gratefulness. Each day focus on three things that you are grateful for. This is a mind-changing practice and is supported by much research.

- Get outdoors in nature and exercise.

- Surround yourself with people of similar values who make you feel uplifted and positive.

- Spend 30 minutes each day breathing and meditating.

- Cut out all processed foods from your diet. I know this is harsh, but trust me, it is necessary for your mental and emotional wellbeing.

- Focus on anti-inflammatory foods and do not consume food that is listed as pro-inflammatory.

- Care for your gut health and microbiome. This is so important, as our microbiome controls everything. Take care of it, so that it can care for you.

- Practise good sleep hygiene.

- Consider supplementation for optimal mind and emotional wellbeing.

'We have the power to choose what we eat, how we sleep, the people we surround ourselves with, and how we choose to show up to life every day.'

Acknowledgements

It seemed such an easy task for someone who loves to write. 'I'll write a book now that I have a little more free time,' I stated with confidence. 'Won't take me long if I just commit. I'll just say no to everything else and spend a month or two writing.' I was completely delusional.

Many thanks to Gareth, Anouska and the team at Exisle Publishing who have worked on this book. I knew from first contact that my book would be in the best hands possible — and I was right. Thanks to Claire de Medici for wonderful editing, encouragement and insights, and Enni Tuomisalo for the design.

Thank you to Jessica Perini for making such helpful suggestions early in the process, and assisting me to bring it all to life.

Thanks to Tiffany Cairns for your beautiful artwork.

Aaron, Jordan, Sue, Helen, Terry, Roma, Jen, Alb, Jillienne, Arthur, Bryce, Juliette, Suzanne, Liam, Jasmine. Thank you for your love and support! And thanks for listening to my constant talk about writing a book to my beautiful friends Penny, Caroline and Shannon.

A heartfelt thanks to my mum. You have always given me so much support and so much love. I hid a lot of what was going on in my mind as that is/was the way I cope, but I always knew you were there for me.

My kids, Lauren and Jared. You saw far more of an unwell mind than I ever wanted you to. I am so blessed to have you, and it's your love that got me through many dark days. Thank you.

And of course Simon my husband, my love. If it wasn't for you I wouldn't have the opportunity or the courage.

Notes

Images

Image of girl smiling on page 154 is from Pixabay.

Preface

1   EA Yeboah (2017). *Toxic in the Mind. Biblica Inc.*

PART 1: BECAUSE WE ARE HUMAN

2   E Easwara (2005). *Words to Live By: Short readings of daily wisdom.* The Blue Mountain Centre of Meditation. p 18.

3   *William James: Writings 1878–1899. The Library of America.* (1992). https://www.loa.org/books/65-writings-1878-1899. Accessed 2019.09.21.

4   Wikisource contributors (2018). The Varieties of Religious Experience: A study in human nature djvu/185, Wikisource, https://en.wikisource.org/w/index.php?title=Page:The_varieties_of_religious_experience,_a_study_in_human_nature.djvu/185&oldid=8450338]. Accessed 2019.10.20.

5   Pursuit of Happiness (2018) https://www.pursuit-of-happiness.org/history-of-happiness/william-james/. Accessed 2019.07.18.

6   B Brown (2010). *The Gifts of Imperfection: Let go of who you think you are supposed to be and embrace who you are.* Hazelden.

7   J Yakeley (2018) 'Shame, Culture and Mental Health.' *Nordic Journal of Psychiatry.* Vol 72 (sup1) pp 20–22. DOI: 10.1080/08039488.2018.1525641

8   Global Burden of Disease Collaborative Network (2017). *Global Burden of Disease Study 2016* (GBD 2016) Results. Seattle, United States: Institute for Health Metrics and Evaluation (IHME). http://ghdx.healthdata.org/gbd-results-tool

9 Many ailments mimic symptoms of mental health disorders. For example thyroid abnormalities are often misdiagnosed as psychiatric disorders. Hypothyroidism leads to fatigue, muscle aches and general malaise.

10 AJ Frances (2012). 'DSM 5 Is Guide Not Bible—Ignore Its Ten Worst Changes. APA approval of DSM-5 is a sad day for psychiatry.' *Psychology Today.* https://www.psychologytoday.com/au/blog/dsm5-in-distress/201212/dsm-5-is-guide-not-bible-ignore-its-ten-worst-changes. Accessed 2019.07.03.

11 AJ Holmes and LM Patrick (2018). 'The Myth of Optimality in Clinical Neuroscience.' *Trends in Cognitive Sciences.* Vol 22 pp 241–57.

12 M Gabriel and V Sharma (2017). 'Antidepressant Discontinuation Syndrome.' *Canadian Medical Association Journal.* Vol 189 (21) p 747. doi:10.1503/cmaj.160991

13 B Liu, J Liu, M Wang et al. (2017) 'From Serotonin to Neuroplasticity: Evolvement of theories for major depressive disorder.' *Frontiers in Cellular Neuroscience.* Vol 11 p 305. https://doi.org/10.3389/fncel.2017.00305

14 A Rush, H Kraemer, H Sackeim et al. (2006). 'Report by the ACNP Task Force on Response and Remission in Major Depressive Disorder.' *Neuropsychopharmacology.* Vol 31 pp 1841–1853. https://doi.org/10.1038/sj.npp.1301131

15 https://www.madinamerica.com/robert-whitaker-new/. Accessed 2019.06.12.

16 AJ Rush, M Trivedi, TJ Carmody, et al. (2004). 'One-year Clinical Outcomes of Depressed Public Sector Outpatients: A benchmark for subsequent studies.' *Biological Psychiatry.* Vol 56 pp 46–53.

17 MA Posternak, DA Solomon, AC Leon et al. (2006). 'The Naturalistic Course of Unipolar Major Depression in the Absence of Somatic Therapy.' *Journal of Nervous and Mental Disease.* Vol 194 pp 324–329.

18 https://kellybroganmd.com/?s=antidepressant+discontinuation. Accessed 2020.02.19.

19 I Kirsch (2014). 'Antidepressants and the Placebo Effect.' *Zeitschrift für Psychologie.* Vol 222 pp 128–134.

20 JC Fournier, RJ DeRubeis, SD Hollon et al. (2010). 'Antidepressant Drug Effects and Depression Severity: A patient-level meta-analysis.' *The Journal of the American Medical Association.* Vol 303 pp 47–53.

21 R Cantrell, AF Young and BC Martin (2002). 'Antibiotic Prescribing in Ambulatory Care Settings for Adults with Colds, Upper Respiratory Tract Infections, and Bronchitis.' *Clinical Therapeutics*. Vol 24 (1) pp 170–182.

22 R Mojtabai (2013). 'Clinician-identified Depression in Community Settings: Concordance with structured-interview diagnoses.' *Psychotherapy and Psychosomatics*. Vol 82 pp 161–69.

23 BL Fredrickson, KM Grewen, KA Coffey, SB Algoe, AM Firestine, JMG Arevalo, SW Cole (2013). 'A Functional Genomic Perspective on Human Well-being.' *Proceedings of the National Academy of Sciences of the United States of America*. Vol 110 pp 13684–13689.

24 A Prat. (2019) 'Nihilism: Friedrich Nietzsche and Nihilism.' *Internet Encyclopedia of Philosophy*. Accessed 2019.09.16.

25 Konow, J., Early, J. (2008). 'The Hedonistic Paradox: Is homo economicus happier?', *Journal of Public Economics*, Vol. 92 (1–2) pp. 1–33.

26 EA Phelps and JE LeDoux (2005). 'Contributions of the Amygdala to Emotion Processing: From animal models to human behavior.' *Neuron*. Vol 48 (2) pp 175–87.

27 WH Jung, S Lee, C Lerman et al. (2018) 'Amygdala Functional and Structural Connectivity Predicts Individual Risk Tolerance'. *Neuron*. Vol 98 (2) pp 394–404.

28 M Gongora, S Teixeira , L Martins et al. (2019.) 'Neurobiological Evidences, Functional and Emotional Aspects Associated with the Amygdala: From "what is it?" to "what's to be done?"' *Neuropsychiatry*. Vol 9 (3) pp 2379–2396.

29 TM Amabile and SJ Kramer (2011). 'The Progress Principle: Using small wins to ignite joy, engagement, and creativity at work.' *Harvard Business Review Press*.

30 Alison Ledgerwood's TED talk on how to reframe setbacks in a positive light is well worth listening to: https://www.npr.org/2019/05/24/725514227/alison-ledgerwood-how-can-we-reframe-setbacks-in-a-positive-light.

31 A Ledgerwood and AE Boydstun (2014). 'Sticky Prospects: Loss frames are cognitively stickier than gain frames.' *Journal of Experimental Psychology*: Genera, doi:10.1037/a0032310

32 M Roser (2018). 'Most of Us are Wrong about How the World has Changed (Especially Those Who are Pessimistic about the Future). Our World in Data' 2018. https://ourworldindata.org/wrong-about-the-world. Accessed 2019.08.13.

33 S Brinson (2018). 'The Psychology of Finding What You're Looking For, Medium.' https://medium.com/s/story/when-blue-becomes-rare-purple-becomes-blue-92472cacce12. Accessed 2019.06.17.

34 Mark Manson (2019). *Everything is Fucked: A book about hope.* Harper Collins.

35 B Specktor (2018). 'Are These Dots Purple, Blue or Proof That Humans Will Never Be Happy?' *Live Science,* https://www.livescience.com/62962-blue-or-purple-dots-illusion.html. Accessed 2019.06.12.

36 C O'Brien (2011). 'Do You Have a Caveman's Brain?' *ASU — Ask A Biologist.* https://askabiologist.asu.edu/plosable/do-you-have-cavemans-brain. Accessed 2020.02.19.

37 A Zalli, O Jovanova, WJG Hoogendijk et al. (2016). 'Low-grade Inflammation Predicts Persistence of Depressive Symptoms.' *Psychopharmacology.* Vol 233 pp 1669–1678; MS Cepeda, P Stang and R Makadia (2016). 'Depression is Associated with High Levels of C-reactive Protein and Low Levels of Fractional Exhaled Nitric Oxide: Results from the 2007–2012 National Health and Nutrition Examination Surveys.' *Journal of Clinical Psychiatry.* Vol 77, pp 1666–1671; BI Goldstein, F Lotrich, DA Axelson et al. (2015). 'Inflammatory Markers Among Adolescents and Young Adults with Bipolar Spectrum Disorders.' *Journal of Clinical Psychiatry.* Vol 76 (11), pp 1556–1563. doi:10.4088/JCP.14m09395.

PART 2: TOOLS TO NOURISH AND PROTECT

38 ND Volkow, GJ Wang, F Telang et al. (2009). 'Inverse Association Between BMI and Prefrontal Metabolic Activity in Healthy Adults.' *Obesity. Vol 17 pp 60–65.*

39 Y Lijun, X Xiaodan, C Gang et al. (2019) 'Inflammation and Decreased Functional Connectivity in a Widely-distributed Network in Depression: Centralized effects in the ventral medial prefrontal cortex.' *Brain, Behavior, and Immunity.* Vol 80 pp 657–666.

40 D Perlmutter and A Perlmutter (2020). *Brain Wash: Detox your mind for clearer thinking, deeper relationships, and lasting happiness.* Yellow Kite Books.

41 JB Miller, N Mann and L Cordain (2009). 'Paleolithic Nutrition: What did our ancestors eat?' *Science School.* http://www.scienceschool.usyd.edu.au/history/2009/media/lectures/4-brand-miller-chapter.pdf. Accessed 2019.07.19.

NOTES

42   The standard American / Australian diet is migrating to other European countries now as well. It is typically low in fibre, high in sugar, sodium and trans fats.

43   MK Zamroziewicz, MT Talukdar, CE Zwilling et al. (2017). 'Nutritional Status, Brain Network Organization, and General Intelligence.' *Neuroimage.* Vol 161 pp 241–250; GY Sun, A Simonyi, KL Fritsche et al. (2018). 'Docosahexaenoic Acid (DHA): An essential nutrient and a nutraceutical for brain health and diseases'. *Prostaglandins, Leukotrienes and Essential Fatty Acids.* Vol 136 pp 3–13; R Gabbianelli and E Damiani (2018). 'Epigenetics and Neurodegeneration: Role of early-life nutrition.' *The Journal of Nutritional Biochemistry.* Vol 57 pp 1–13.

44   G Adshead (2017). 'Antidepressants and Murder: Case not closed.' *British Medical Journal.* Vol 358 p 3697. doi:10.1136 / bmj.j3697 pmid:28768656

45   R Whitaker (2010). *Anatomy of an Epidemic: Magic bullets, psychiatric drugs, and the astonishing rise of mental illness in America.* Broadway Books; Northwestern University (2009). 'Why Antidepressants Don't Work For So Many.' *ScienceDaily.* www.sciencedaily.com / releases / 2009 / 10 / 091023163346.htm. Accessed 2019.06.16.

46   AE Tufan, R Bilici, G Usta et al. (2012). 'Mood Disorder with Mixed, Psychotic Features Due to Vitamin B12 Deficiency in an Adolescent: Case report.' *Child and Adolescent Psychiatry and Mental health.* Vol 6 (1) p 25. doi:10.1186 / 1753-2000-6-25; N Jayaram, MG Rao, A Narasimha et al. (2013) 'Vitamin B(1)(2) Levels and Psychiatric Symptomatology: A case series.' *Journal of Neuropsychiatry and Clinical Neurosciences.* Vol 25 (2) pp 150–152.

47   M Valles-Colomer, G Falony, Y Darzi et al. (2019). 'The Neuroactive Potential of the Human Gut Microbiota in Quality of Life and Depression.' *Nature Microbiology.* doi: 10.1038 / s41564-018-0337-x [Epub ahead of print].

48   BJ Kaplan, JJ Rucklidge, A Romijn et al. (2015). 'The Emerging Field of Nutritional Mental Health: Inflammation, the microbiome, oxidative stress, and mitochondrial function.' *Clinical Psychological Science.* Vol 3 (6) pp 964–980; R Alam, HM Abdolmaleky and JR Zhou (2017). 'Microbiome, Inflammation, Epigenetic Alterations, and Mental Diseases.' *American Journal of Medical Genetics Part B.* Vol 174B pp 651–660.

49   L Cordain, S Boyd Eaton, A Sebastian et al. (2005) 'Origins and Evolution of the Western Diet: Health implications for the 21st century.' *The American Journal of Clinical Nutrition.* Vol 81 (2) p 341 https:// doi.org / 10.1093 / ajcn.81.2.341

50 Q Chang, W Wang, G Regev-Yochay et al. (2015). 'Antibiotics in Agriculture and the Risk to Human Health: How worried should we be?' *Evolutionary Applications*. Vol 8 (3) pp 240–247. doi:10.1111/eva.12185

51 ND Volkow, GJ Wang, JS Fowler et al. (2011) 'Food and Drug Reward: Overlapping circuits in human obesity and addiction.' In: C Carter and J Dalley (eds) *Brain Imaging in Behavioral Neuroscience*. Current Topics in Behavioral Neuroscience. Vol 11. Springer.

52 L Lucas, L Riddell, G Liem et al. (2010) 'The Influence of Sodium on Liking and Consumption of Salty Food.' *Journal of Food Science*. Vol 76 (1) pp. 72–76.

53 Information about the Deakin University Food and Mood Centre. https://foodandmoodcentre.com.au/about/. Accessed 2019.06.24.

54 FN Jacka , A Mykletun, M Berk et al. (2011). 'The Association between Habitual Diet Quality and the Common Mental Disorders in Community-dwelling Adults: The Hordaland Health Study.' *Psychosomatic Medicine*. Vol 73 pp 483–490; FN Jacka, JA Pasco, A Mykletun et al. (2010) 'Association of Western and Traditional Diets with Depression and Anxiety in Women.' *American Journal of Psychiatry*. Vol 167 pp 305–311.

55 T Sergentanis, D Panagiotakos, I Sergentanis et al. (2013). 'Mediterranean Diet, Stroke, Cognitive Impairment, and Depression: A meta-analysis.' *Annals of Neurology*. Vol 74. 10.1002/ana.23944

56 N Parletta, D Zarnowiecki, J Cho et al. (2019). 'A Mediterranean-style Dietary Intervention Supplemented with Fish Oil Improves Diet Quality and Mental Health in People with Depression: A randomized controlled trial (HELFIMED)', *Nutritional Neuroscience*. Vol 22 (7) pp 474–487.

57 LS Abdelli, A Samsam and SA Naser (2019). 'Propionic Acid Induces Gliosis and Neuro-inflammation Through Modulation of PTEN/AKT Pathway in Autism Spectrum Disorder.' *Scientific Reports*. Vol 9. https://doi.org/10.1038/s41598-019-45348-z.

58 FN Jacka, N Cherbuin, K Janstey et al. (2015). 'Western Diet is Associated with a Smaller Hippocampus: A longitudinal investigation.' *BMC Medicine*. Vol 13 p 215.

59 FN Jacka, A O'Neil, R Opie et al. (2017). 'A Randomised Controlled Trial of Dietary Improvement for Adults with Major Depression (the 'SMILES' trial).' *BMC Medicine*. Vol 15 pp 23.

60 JS Lai, S Hiles, A Bisquera et al. (2013). 'A Systematic Review and Meta-analysis of Dietary Patterns and Depression in Community-dwelling Adults.' *American Journal of Clinical Nutrition*. Vol 99 (1) pp 181–97.

61 SE McMartin, FN Jacka and I Colman (2013) 'The Association Between Fruit and Vegetable Consumption and Mental Health Disorders: Evidence from five waves of a national survey of Canadians.' *Preventive Medicine*. Vol 56 (3) pp 225–230.

62 N Wahls (2014). 'About the Wahls Protocol' https://terrywahls.com/about-the-wahls-protocol/. Accessed 2019.06.24.

63 https://www.thepages.com.bd/2019/07/07/from-bed-ridden-to-biking-meet-the-woman-who-tackled-ms-with-diet/. Accessed 2019.06.24.

64 S Thongprakaisang, A Thiantanawat, N Rangkadilok et al. (2013) 'Glyphosate Induces Human Breast Cancer Cells Growth Via Estrogen Receptors.' *Food and Chemical Toxicology*. Vol 59 pp 129–136.

65 C Jayasumana, P Paranagama, S Agampodi et al. (2015). 'Drinking Well Water and Occupational Exposure to Herbicides is Associated with Chronic Kidney Disease.' In Padavi-Sripura. *Sri Lanka Environmental Health*. Vol 14 (1) p 6.

66 C Sakpa and S Popoola (2018). 'Effects of Glyphosate on Sperm Parameters and Pregnancy Success Rate in Wistar Rats.' *Annals of Biomedical Sciences*. Vol 17 (2), pp 156–164.

67 Z Honeycutt and H Rowlands (2014). 'Glyphosate Testing Report: Findings in American mothers' breast milk, urine and water.' *Moms Across America*. http://www.momsacrossamerica.com/glyphosate_testing_results. Accessed 2019.07.15.

68 R Di Cagno, CG Rizzello, M De Angelis et al. (2008). 'Use of Selected Sourdough Strains of Lactobacillus for Removing Gluten and Enhancing the Nutritional Properties of Gluten-free Bread.' *Journal of Food Protection*. Vol 71 pp 1491–1495. doi: 10.4315/0362-028X-71.7.1491

69 HW Lopez, V Krespine, C Guy et al. (2001). 'Prolonged Fermentation of Whole Wheat Sourdough Reduces Phytate Level and Increases Soluble Magnesium.' *Journal of Agricultural and Food Chemistry*. Vol 49 (5), pp 2657–2662.

70 B Chassaing, O Koren, JK Goodrich et al. (2015). 'Dietary Emulsifiers Impact the Mouse Gut Microbiota Promoting Colitis and Metabolic Syndrome.' *Nature*. Vol 519 (7541) pp 92–96. doi:10.1038/nature14232

71 SAE Peters, E Dunford, A Jones et al. (2017). 'Incorporating Added Sugar Improves the Performance of the Health Star Rating Front-of-Pack Labelling System in Australia. *Nutrients*. Vol 9 p 701.

72 E Benny (2012). 'Natural Modifications: The FDA's need to promulgate an official definition of "natural" that includes genetically modified organisms.' *George Washington Law Review Arguendo*. Vol 80 (5) pp 1504–1526.

73 MLFernandez (2006). 'Dietary Cholesterol Provided by Eggs and Plasma Lipoproteins in Healthy Populations'. *Current Opinion in Clinical Nutrition and Metabolic Care*. Vol 9 (1) pp 8–12. doi:10.1097/01.mco.0000171152.51034.bf

74 JA Welsh , A Sharma, JL Abramson et al. (2010). 'Caloric Sweetener Consumption and Dyslipidemia Among US Adults.' *The Journal of the American Medical Association*. Vol 303 (15) pp 1490–1497. doi:10.1001/jama.2010.449

75 RP Mensink and M Katan (1990). 'Effect of Dietary Trans Fatty Acids on High-density and Low-density Lipoprotein Cholesterol Levels in Healthy Subjects.' *New England Journal of Medicine*. Vol 323 (7) pp 439–445.

76 https://www.fda.gov/food/chemicals/survey-data-acrylamide-food. Accessed 2019.08.12.

77 IJ Skypala, M Williams, L Reeves et al. (2015). 'Sensitivity to Food Additives, Vaso-active Amines and Salicylates: A review of the evidence.' *Clinical and Translational Allergy*. Vol 5 p 34 doi:10.1186/s13601-015-0078-3

78 http://www.foodstandards.gov.au/consumer/additives/additivecontrol/Pages/default.aspx. Accessed 2019. 08.14; https://daa.asn.au/smart-eating-for-you/smart-eating-fast-facts/children/can-food-additives-affect-my-childs-behaviour/. Accessed 2019.08.14.

79 AN Payne, C Chassard and C Lacroix (2012). 'Gut Microbial Adaptation to Dietary Consumption of Fructose, Artificial Sweeteners and Sugar Alcohols: Implications for host–microbe interactions contributing to obesity.' *Obesity Reviews*. Vol 13 pp 799–809; A Agus, J Denizot, J Thévenot et al. (2015). 'Western Diet Induces a Shift in Microbiota Composition Enhancing Susceptibility to Adherent-invasive E. coli Infection and Intestinal Inflammation.' *Scientific Reports*. Vol 6: 19032.10.1038/srep19032

80 L Hrncirova, T Hudcovic, E Sukova et al. (2019). 'Human Gut Microbes are Susceptible to Antimicrobial Food Additives in Vitro.' *Folia Microbiologica* (Praha). Vol 32 pp 99–103.

81 MK Holder, NV Peters, J Whylings et al. (2019). 'Dietary Emulsifiers Consumption Alters Anxiety-like and Social-related Behaviors in Mice in a Sex-dependent Manner.' *Scientific Reports*. Vol 9 p 172. https://doi.org/10.1038/s41598-018-36890-3

82 I Freckelton (2005). 'Madhouse: A tragic tale of megalomania and modern medicine' (Book review). *Psychiatry, Psychology and Law*. Vol 12 (2) pp 435–438.

83 T Canli (2014). 'Reconceptualizing Major Depressive Disorder as an Infectious Disease.' *Biology of Mood & Anxiety Disorders*. Vol 4, p 10. doi:10.1186/2045-5380-4-10

84 RE Baynes, KJ Dix and JE Riviere (2001). 'Chapter 6: Distribution and Pharmacokinetics Models.' **This chapter was editorially abbreviated and reformatted from KJ Dix (2001). 'Absorption, Distribution and Pharmacokinetics', Chapter 24 in *Handbook of Pesticide Toxicology* (R Krieger, Ed.), 2nd edition, Academic Press.

85 S Cahalan (2013). *Brain on Fire: My month of madness*. Simon and Schuster.

86 I Kirsch (2014). 'Antidepressants and the Placebo Effect.' *Zeitschrift fur Psychologie*. Vol 222 (3), pp 128–134. doi:10.1027/2151-2604/a000176

87 I Labuschagne, K L Phan, A Wood et al. (2010). 'Oxytocin Attenuates Amygdala Reactivity to Fear in Generalized Social Anxiety Disorder.' *Neuropsychopharmacology*. Vol 35(12) pp 2403–2413. https://doi.org/10.1038/npp.2010.123

88 H Costa, TA Gonçalves and M Oliveira (2018). '3-MCPD Occurrence in Vegetable Oils: Impact on human nutrition and future challenges.' *EC Nutrition*. Vol 13 (7) pp 455–469.

89 CY Ng, Y Kamisah, O Faizah et al. (2012). 'The Role of Repeatedly Heated Soybean Oil in the Development of Hypertension in Rats: Association with vascular inflammation.' *International Journal of Experimental Pathology*. Vol 93 (5) pp 377–387. doi:10.1111/j.1365-2613.2012.00839.x

90 E Patterson, R Wall, GF Fitzgerald et al. (2012). 'Health Implications of High Dietary Omega-6 Polyunsaturated Fatty Acids.' *Journal of Nutrition and Metabolism*. Vol 2012; 539426. doi:10.1155/2012/539426

91 A Sánchez-Villegas, L Verberne, J De Irala et al. (2011). 'Dietary Fat Intake and the Risk of Depression: The SUN Project.' *PloS one.* Vol 6 (1) pp 162–168 doi:10.1371/journal.pone.0016268

92 BA Golomb, MA Evans, HL White et al (2012). 'Trans Fat Consumption and Aggression.' *PloS one.* Vol 7 (3). doi:10.1371/journal.pone.0032175

93 PA Ford, K Jaceldo-Siegl, JW Lee et al. (2016). 'Trans Fatty Acid Intake is Related to Emotional Affect in the Adventist Health Study-2.' *Nutrition Research.* Vol 36 (6), pp 509–517. doi:10.1016/j.nutres.2016.01.005

94 I Aeberli, PA Gerber, M Hochuli et al. (2011). 'Low to Moderate Sugar-sweetened Beverage Consumption Impairs Glucose and Lipid Metabolism and Promotes Inflammation in Healthy Young Men: A randomized controlled trial.' *The American Journal of Clinical Nutrition.* Vol 94 (2) pp 479–485, https://doi.org/10.3945/ajcn.111.013540

95 NA Harrison, L Brydon, C Walker et al. (2009). 'Inflammation Causes Mood Changes Through Alterations in Subgenual Cingulate Activity and Mesolimbic Connectivity.' *Biological Psychiatry.* Vol 66 (5) pp 407–414.

96 S Wilson (2014). *I Quit Sugar. The complete 8-week program.* Pan Macmillan.

97 A Sawani, M Farhangi, AN Chandrakala et al. (2018). 'Limiting Dietary Sugar Improves Pediatric Sinonasal Symptoms and Reduces Inflammation.' *Journal of Medicinal Food.* Vol 21 (6) http://doi.org/10.1089/jmf.2017.012

98 I Garcia-Mantrana, M Selma-Royo, C Alcantara et al. (2018). 'Shifts on Gut Microbiota Associated to Mediterranean Diet Adherence and Specific Dietary Intakes on General Adult Population.' *Frontiers in Microbiology.* Vol 9 p 890. doi:10.3389/fmicb.2018.00890

99 Y Cho, D Kim, W Seo et al. (2019). 'Fructose Promotes Leaky Gut, Endotoxemia, and Liver Fibrosis Through Ethanol-Inducible Cytochrome P450-2E1–Mediated Oxidative and Nitrative Stress.' *Hepatology.* doi:10.1002/hep.30652

100 M Berk, LJ Williams, FN Jacka et al. (2013). 'So Depression is an Inflammatory Disease, But Where Does the Inflammation Come From?' *BMC Medicine.* Vol 11, p 200. doi:10.1186/1741-7015-11-200; M Maes, M Kubera and JC Leunis. (2008). 'The Gut–Brain Barrier in Major Depression: Intestinal mucosal dysfunction with an increased translocation of LPS from gram negative enterobacteria (leaky gut) plays

a role in the inflammatory pathophysiology of depression.' *Neuroendocrinology Letters*. Vol 29 (1) pp 117–124.

101 E Lopez-Garcia, MB Schulze, TT Fung et al. (2004). 'Major Dietary Patterns are Related to Plasma Concentrations of Markers of Inflammation and Endothelial Dysfunction.' *The American Journal of Clinical Nutrition*. Vol 80 (4) pp 1029–1035, https://doi.org/10.1093/ajcn/80.4.1029

102 JC Antvorskov, P Fundova, K Buschard et al. (2013), 'Dietary Gluten Alters the Balance of Pro-inflammatory and Anti-inflammatory Cytokines in T Cells of BALB/c Mice.' *Immunology*. Vol 138 pp 23-33. doi:10.1111/imm.12007; AM Henschel, SM Cabrera, ML Kaldunski et al.(2018). 'Modulation of the Diet and Gastrointestinal Microbiota Normalizes Systemic Inflammation and β-cell Chemokine Expression Associated with Autoimmune Diabetes Susceptibility.' *PloS one*. Vol 13 (1), e0190351. doi:10.1371/journal.pone.0190351.

103 D Perlmutter (2010). 'Gluten Sensitivity and the Impact on the Brain' *HuffPost*. https://www.huffingtonpost.com/dr-david-perlmutter-md/gluten-impacts-the-brain_b_785901.html. Accessed 2019.09.27

104 M Hadjivassiliou, A Gibson, GB Davies-Jones et al. (1996). 'Does Cryptic Gluten Sensitivity Play a Part in Neurological Illness?' *The Lancet*. Vol 347 (8998) pp 369–371.

105 S Peters, J Muir and P Gibson (2014). 'Gluten Sensitivity Without Coeliac Disease — A new twist.' *Agro Food Industry Hi-Tech*. Vol 25 pp 38–42.

106 JK Kiecolt-Glaser, MA Belury, R Andridge et al. (2011). 'Omega-3 Supplementation Lowers Inflammation and Anxiety in Medical Students: A randomized controlled trial.' *Brain, Behavior, and Immunity*. Vol 25 (8) pp 1725–1734; T Larrieu, S Layé (2018). 'Food for Mood: Relevance of nutritional omega-3 fatty acids for depression and anxiety.' *Frontiers in Physiology*. Vol 9 p 1047. doi:10.3389/fphys.2018.01047; K Su, P Tseng, P Lin et al. (2018). 'Association of Use of Omega-3 Polyunsaturated Fatty Acids With Changes in Severity of Anxiety Symptoms: A systematic review and meta-analysis.' *The Journal of the American Medical Association*. Vol 1 (5), e182327. doi:10.1001/jamanetworkopen.2018.2327.

107 G Grosso, F Galvano, S Marventano et al. (2014). 'Omega-3 Fatty Acids and Depression: Scientific evidence and biological mechanisms.' *Oxidative Medicine and Cellular Longevity*. Vol 313570. doi:10.1155/2014/313570

[108] E Prato and F Biandolin (2015). 'Chapter 16: The Contribution of Fish to the Mediterranean Diet.' In VR Preedy and RR Watson (eds), *The Mediterranean Diet*, Academic Press, pp 165–174.

[109] C Lassale, GD Batty, A Baghdadli et al. (2019). 'Healthy Dietary Indices and Risk of Depressive Outcomes: A systematic review and meta-analysis of observational studies.' *Molecular Psychiatry*. Vol 24 pp 965–986.

[110] L Parkinson and R Keast (2014). 'Oleocanthal, a Phenolic Derived from Virgin Olive Oil: A review of the beneficial effects on inflammatory disease.' *International Journal of Molecular Science*. Vol 15 pp 12323–12334; L Parkinson and S Cicerale (2016). 'The Health Benefiting Mechanisms of Virgin Olive Oil Phenolic Compounds.' *Molecules* (Basel, Switzerland). Vol 21 (12) pp 1734. doi:10.3390/molecules21121734

[111] R Chowdhury, S Warnakula, S Kunutsor et al. (2014). 'Association of Dietary, Circulating, and Supplement Fatty Acids With Coronary Risk: A systematic review and meta-analysis.' *Annals of Internal Medicine*. Vol 160 pp 398–406. doi: 10.7326/M13-1788; CE Ramsden, D Zamora, S Majchrzak-Hong et al.(2016). 'Re-evaluation of the Traditional Diet–Heart Hypothesis: Analysis of recovered data from Minnesota Coronary Experiment (1968–73).' *British Medical Journal (Clinical research ed.)*. Vol 353 p 1246. doi:10.1136/bmj.i1246

[112] JJ DiNicolantonio (2014). 'The Cardiometabolic Consequences of Replacing Saturated Fats with Carbohydrates or Ω-6 Polyunsaturated Fats: Do the dietary guidelines have it wrong?' *Open Heart*. Vol 1 (1): e000032. doi: 10.1136/openhrt-2013-000032

[113] WMM Verschuren, DR Jacobs, BPM Bloemberg et al. (1995). 'Serum Total Cholesterol and Long-term Coronary Heart Disease Mortality in Different Cultures. Twenty-five year follow-up of the Seven Countries Study.' *The Journal of the American Medical Association*. Vol 274 pp 131–136.

[114] NJ Temple (2018). 'Fat, Sugar, Whole Grains and Heart Disease: 50 years of confusion.' *Nutrients*. Vol 10 (1) p 39. doi:10.3390/nu10010039

[115] SV Joseph, I Edirisinghe and BM Burton-Freeman (2014). 'Berries: Anti-inflammatory effects in humans.' *Journal of Agricultural and Food Chemistry*. Vol 62 (18), pp 3886–3903 DOI: 10.1021/jf4044056; B Yang and M Kortesniemi (2015). 'Clinical Evidence on Potential Health Benefits of Berries.' *Current Opinion in Food Science*. Vol 2 pp 36–42.

[116] A Basu, M Foster, N Betts et al. (2016). 'Effects of Dietary Strawberries on Inflammatory Biomarkers in Participants with Abdominal Obesity and Dyslipidemia.' *The FASEB Journal*. Vol 30 (1) supplement 1174.10-1174.10

[117] N Ocean, P Howley and J Ensor (2019). 'Lettuce be Happy: A longitudinal UK study on the relationship between fruit and vegetable consumption and well-being.' *Social Science & Medicine*. Vol 222 pp 335–345; R Mujcic and A J Oswald (2016). 'Evolution of Well-Being and Happiness After Increases in Consumption of Fruit and Vegetables.' *American Journal of Public Health*. Vol 106 pp 1504–1510.

[118] T Wahls and E Adamson (2015). *The Wahls Protocol*. Vermilion.

[119] CA Lang, BJ Mills, HL Lang et al. (2002). 'High Blood Glutathione Levels Accompany Excellent Physical and Mental Health in Women Ages 60 to 103 Years.' *Journal of Laboratory and Clinical Medicine*. Vol 140 (6) pp 413–417.

[120] CY Chang, DS Ke and JY Chen. (2009). 'Essential Fatty Acids and Human Brain.' *Acta Neurologica Taiwanica*. Vol 18 (4) pp 231–241.

[121] SJ Hewlings and DS Kalman (2017). 'Curcumin: A review of its effects on human health.' *Foods (Basel, Switzerland)*. Vol 6 (10) p 92. doi:10.3390/foods6100092

[122] A Wu, EE Noble, E Tyagi et al. (2015). 'Curcumin Boosts DHA in the Brain: Implications for the prevention of anxiety disorders.' *Biochimica et Biophysica Acta*. Vol 1852 (5) pp 951–961.

[123] J Sanmukhani, V Satodia, J Trivedi et al. (2014). 'Efficacy and Safety of Curcumin in Major Depressive Disorder: A randomized controlled trial.' *Phytotherapy Research*. Vol 28 pp 579–585. doi:10.1002/ptr.5025

[124] H Esmaily, A Sahebkar, M Iranshahi et al. (2015). 'An Investigation of the Effects of Curcumin on Anxiety and Depression in Obese Individuals: A randomized controlled trial.' *Chinese Journal of Integrative Medicine*. Vol 21 pp 332–338.

[125] Peterson, C. T., Vaughn, A. R., Sharma, V., Chopra, D., Mills, P. J., Peterson, S. N., & Sivamani, R. K. (2018). 'Effects of Turmeric and Curcumin Dietary Supplementation on Human Gut Microbiota: A double-blind, randomized, placebo-controlled pilot study.' *Journal of Evidence-based Integrative Medicine*, 23, 2515690X18790725. https://doi.org/10.1177/2515690X18790725

[126] SC Bischoff (2010). 'Gut Health: A new objective in medicine?' *BMC Medicine*. Vol 9 p 24. 10.1186/1741-7015-9-24.

[127] JR Kelly, PJ Kennedy, JF Cryan et al. (2015). 'Breaking Down the Barriers: The gut microbiome, intestinal permeability and stress-related psychiatric disorders.' *Frontiers in Cellular Neuroscience*. Vol 9 p 392. doi:10.3389/fncel.2015.00392

[128] I Ezkurdia, D Juan, JM Rodriguez et al. (2013). 'The Shrinking Human Protein Coding Complement: Are there now fewer than 20,000 genes?' https://arxiv.org/abs/1312.7111. Accessed 2019.09.03.

[129] S Gondalia, L Parkinson, C Stough et al. (2019). 'Gut Microbiota and Bipolar Disorder: A review of mechanisms and potential targets for adjunctive therapy.' *Psychopharmacology*. Vol 236 (5) p 1433. https://doi.org/10.1007/s00213-019-05248-6

[130] N Sudo, Y Chida, Y Aiba et al. (2004). 'Postnatal Microbial Colonization Programs: The hypothalamic–pituitary–adrenal system for stress response in mice.' *The Journal of Physiology*. Vol 558 pp 263–275. doi:10.1113/jphysiol.2004.063388

[131] E Young (2012). 'Gut Instincts: The secrets of your second brain.' *New Scientist*. https://www.newscientist.com/article/mg21628951.900-gut-instincts-the-secrets-of-your-second-brain. Accessed 2019.08.24

[132] A Hart and MA Kamm (2002). 'Mechanisms of Initiation and Perpetuation of Gut Inflammation by Stress.' *Alimentary Pharmacology & Therapeutics*. Vol 16 pp 2017–2028; V Leccioli, M Oliveri, M Romeo et al. (2017). 'A New Proposal for the Pathogenic Mechanism of Non-coeliac/Non-allergic Gluten/Wheat Sensitivity: Piecing together the puzzle of recent scientific evidence.' *Nutrients*. Vol 9 (11) p 1203.

[133] K Lange, M Buerger, A Stallmach et al. (2016). 'Effects of Antibiotics on Gut Microbiota.' *Digestive Diseases*. Vol 34 pp 260–268. doi: 10.1159/000443360; C Gustafson (2016). 'Inflammation in the Gut Drives Systemic Inflammation.' *Integrative Medicine*. Vol 15 (4) pp 32–34; AP Bhatt, DB Gunasekara, J Speer et al. (2018). 'Nonsteroidal Anti-Inflammatory Drug-Induced Leaky Gut Modeled Using Polarized Monolayers of Primary Human Intestinal Epithelial Cells.' *ACS Infectious Diseases*. Vol 4 (1) pp 46–52. doi:10.1021/acsinfecdis.7b00139

[134] I Bjarnason, A MacPherson and D Hollander (1995). 'Intestinal Permeability: An overview.' *Gastroenterology*. Vol 108 pp 1566–1581.

[135] S Breit, A Kupferberg, G Rogler et al. (2018). 'Vagus Nerve as Modulator of the Brain–Gut Axis in Psychiatric and Inflammatory Disorders.' *Frontiers in Psychiatry*. Vol 9 p 44. doi:10.3389/fpsyt.2018.00044

136 Q Mu, VJ Tavella and XM Luo (2018). 'Role of *Lactobacillus reuteri* in Human Health and Diseases.' *Frontiers in Microbiology*. Vol 9 p 757. doi:10.3389/ fmicb.2018.00757

137 M Sgritta, S Dooling, S Buffington et al. (2018). 'Mechanisms Underlying Microbial-Mediated Changes in Social Behavior in Mouse Models of Autism Spectrum Disorder.' *Neuron*. 101. 10.1016/j.neuron.11.018

138 S Panda, I El khader F Casellas et al. (2014). 'Short-Term Effect of Antibiotics on Human Gut Microbiota.' *PLoS ONE*. Vol 9 (4): e95476. https://doi.org/10.1371/ journal.pone.0095476

139 O Köhler-Forsberg, L Petersen, C Gasse et al. (2018). 'A Nationwide Study in Denmark of the Association Between Treated Infections and the Subsequent Risk of Treated Mental Disorders in Children and Adolescents'. *JAMA Psychiatry*. Vol 76 (3) pp 271–279. doi:10.1001/jamapsychiatry.2018.3428

140 C Jernberg, S Lofmark, C Edlund et al. (2007). 'Long-term Ecological Impacts of Antibiotic Administration on the Human Intestinal Microbiota'. *ISME Journal*. Vol 1 pp 56–66.

141 G Reid (2016). 'Probiotics: Definition, scope and mechanisms of action.' *Best Practice & Research Clinical Gastroenterology*. Vol 30 (1) pp 17–25; F Jabr (2017). 'Probiotics are No Panacea.' *Scientific American*. Vol 317 (1) pp 26–27. doi:10.1038/ scientificamerican0717-26

142 B Corthésy, HR Gaskins and A Mercenier (2007). 'Cross-Talk between Probiotic Bacteria and the Host Immune System.' *The Journal of Nutrition*. Vol 137 (3) pp 781S–790S.

143 M Messaoudi, N Violle, J Bisson et al. (2011). 'Beneficial Psychological Effects of a Probiotic Formulation (*Lactobacillus helveticus R0052* and *Bifidobacterium longum R0175)* in Healthy Human Volunteers.' *Gut Microbes*. Vol 2 (4) pp 256–261; S Weston, A Halbert, P Richmond et al. (2005). 'Effects of Probiotics on Atopic Dermatitis: A randomised controlled trial.' *Archives of Disease in Childhood*. Vol 90 pp 892-897; R Huang, K Wang and J Hu (2016). 'Effect of Probiotics on Depression: A systematic review and meta-analysis of randomized controlled trials.' *Nutrients*. Vol 8 (8), pp 483. doi:10.3390/nu8080483.

144 HA Hong, LH Duc, SM Cutting. (2005). 'The Use of Bacterial Spore Formers as Probiotics.' *FEMS Microbiology Reviews*. Vol 29 (4) pp 813–835. https://doi. org/10.1016/j.femsre.2004.12.001

[145] BK McFarlin, AL Henning, EM Bowman et al. (2017). 'Oral Spore-based Probiotic Supplementation was Associated with Reduced Incidence of Post-prandial Dietary Endotoxin, Triglycerides, and Disease Risk Biomarkers.' *World Journal of Gastrointestinal Pathophysiology*. Vol 8 (3) pp 117–126.

[146] L Steenbergen, R Sellaro, S van Hemert et al (2015). 'A Randomized Controlled Trial to Test the Effect of Multispecies Probiotics on Cognitive Reactivity to Sad Mood.' *Brain, Behavior, and Immunity*. Vol 48 pp 258–264.

[147] M Pirbaglou, J Katz, RJ de Souza et al. (2016). 'Probiotic Supplementation Can Positively Affect Anxiety and Depressive Symptoms: A systematic review of randomized controlled trials.' *Nutrition Research* 36 (9) pp 889–98; A Bharwani, MF Mian, MG Surette et al. (2017). 'Oral Treatment with *Lactobacillus rhamnosus* Attenuates Behavioural Deficits and Immune Changes in Chronic Social Stress.' *BMC Medicine*. Vol 15 (1) p 7.

[148] E Williams Barnhardt, M Jacque and TR Sharma (2016). 'Brief Reversible Psychosis and Altered Mental Status in a Patient With Folate Deficiency: A case report.' *The Primary Care Companion for CNS disorders*. Vol 18 (1) 10.4088/PCC.15l01839. doi:10.4088/PCC.15l01839; TS Rao, MR Asha, BN Ramesh et al. (2008). 'Understanding Nutrition, Depression and Mental Illnesses.' *Indian Journal of Psychiatry*. Vol 50 (2) pp 77–82. doi:10.4103/0019-5545.42391

[149] A Coppen and C Bolander-Gouaille (2005). 'Treatment of Depression: Time to consider folic acid and vitamin B12.' *Journal of Psychopharmacology*. Vol 19 (1) pp 59–65; M Bičíková, M Dušková, J Vítků et al. (2015). 'Vitamin D in Anxiety and Affective Disorders.' *Physiological Research*. Vol 64 (Suppl 2): S101–3

[150] A Cuomo, G Maina, S Bolognesi, et al (2019) 'Prevalence and Correlates of Vitamin D Deficiency in a Sample of 290 Inpatients With Mental Illness.' *Front Psychiatry*. Vol 10, p 167.

[151] JH Cunningham, G Milligan and L Trevisan (2001). 'Minerals in Australian Fruits and Vegetables — A comparison of levels between the 1980s and 2000.' *Food Standards Australia New Zealand*

[152] SK Duckett, JPS Neel, JP Fontenot et al. (2009). 'Effects of Winter Stocker Growth Rate and Finishing System On: III. Tissue Proximate, Fatty Acid, Vitamin, and Cholesterol Content.' *Journal of Animal Science*. Vol 87 (9) pp 2961–2970.

153 J Zemdegs, Q Rainer, CP Grossmann et al. (2018). 'Anxiolytic- and Antidepressant-like Effects of Fish Oil-enriched Diet in Brain-derived Neurotrophic Factor Deficient Mice.' *Frontiers in Neuroscience*. Vol 201 p 974.

154 K Kitajka, AJ Sinclair, RS Weisinger et al. (2004). 'Effects of Dietary Omega-3 Polyunsaturated Fatty Acids on Brain Gene Expression.' *Proceedings of the National Academy of Sciences of the United States of America*. Vol 101 (30) pp 10931–10936. doi:10.1073/pnas.0402342101

155 OI Okereke, CF Reynolds, D Mischoulon et al. (2018). 'The VITamin D and OmegA-3 TriaL-Depression Endpoint Prevention (VITAL-DEP): Rationale and design of a large-scale ancillary study evaluating vitamin D and marine omega-3 fatty acid supplements for prevention of late-life depression.' *Contemporary Clinical Trials*. Vol 68 pp 133–145.

156 VR Ramprasath, I Eyal, S Zchut et al. (2013). 'Enhanced Increase of Omega-3 Index in Healthy Individuals with Response to 4-week n-3 Fatty Acid Supplementation From Krill Oil Versus Fish Oil.' *Lipids in Health and Disease*. Vol 12 p 178. doi:10.1186/1476-511X-12-178

157 K Yurko-Mauro, J Kralovec, E Bailey-Hall et al. (2015). 'Similar Eicosapentaenoic Acid and Docosahexaenoic Acid Plasma Levels Achieved With Fish Oil or Krill Oil in a Randomized Double-blind Four-week Bioavailability Study.' *Lipids in Health and Disease*. Vol 1 p 99. doi:10.1186/s12944-015-0109-z

158 AL Dawson, S Kawaguchi, CK King et al. (2018). 'Turning Microplastics into Nanoplastics Through Digestive Fragmentation by Antarctic Krill.' *Nature Communications*. Vol 9 p 1001. doi: 10.1038/s41467-018-03465-9

159 A Coppen and C Bolander-Gouaille (2005). 'Treatment of Depression: Time to consider folic acid and vitamin B12.' *Journal of Psychopharmacology*. Vol 19 (1) pp 59–65.

160 WJH Brenda, J Penninx, L Guralnik et al. (2000). 'Vitamin B12 Deficiency and Depression in Physically Disabled Older Women: Epidemiologic evidence from the women's health and aging study.' *American Journal of Psychiatry*. Vol 157 (5) pp 715–721.

161 WJ Walsh. (2014). *Nutrient Power: Heal your biochemistry and heal your brain.* Skyhorse Publishing.

[162] R Anglin, Z Samaan, S Walter et al. (2013). 'Vitamin D Deficiency and Depression in Adults: Systematic review and meta-analysis.' *British Journal of Psychiatry*. Vol 202 (2) pp 100–107. doi:10.1192/bjp.bp.111.106666

[163] WJG Hoogendijk, P Lips, MG Dik et al. (2008). 'Depression is Associated With Decreased 25-Hydroxyvitamin D and Increased Parathyroid Hormone Levels in Older Adults.' *Archives of General Psychiatry*. Vol 65 (5) pp 508–512. doi:10.1001/archpsyc.65.5.508; R Vieth, S Kimball, A Hu et al. (2004). 'Randomized Comparison of the Effects of the Vitamin D3 Adequate Intake Versus 100 mcg (4000 IU) Per Day on Biochemical Responses and the Wellbeing of Patients.' *Nutrition Journal*. Vol 3 p 8. doi:10.1186/1475-2891-3-8; CH Wilkins, YI Sheline, CM Roe et al. (2006). 'Vitamin D Deficiency is Associated With Low Mood and Worse Cognitive Performance in Older Adults.' *The American Journal of Geriatric Psychiatry*. Vol 14 (12) pp 1032–1040.

[164] S Fazelian, R Amani, Z Paknahad et al. (2019). 'Effect of Vitamin D Supplement on Mood Status and Inflammation in Vitamin D Deficient Type 2 Diabetic Women with Anxiety: A randomized clinical trial.' *International Journal of Preventive Medicine*. Vol 10 p 17. doi:10.4103/ijpvm.IJPVM_174_18

[165] HM Trang, DE Cole, LA Rubin et al. (1998). 'Evidence that Vitamin D3 Increases Serum 25-hydroxyvitamin D More Efficiently Than Does Vitamin D2.' *The American Journal of Clinical Nutrition*. Vol 68 (4) pp 854–858, https://doi.org/10.1093/ajcn/68.4.854; L Tripkovic, H Lambert, K Hart et al. (2012). 'Comparison of Vitamin D2 and Vitamin D3 Supplementation in Raising Serum 25-hydroxyvitamin D Status: A systematic review and meta-analysis.' *The American Journal of Clinical Nutrition*. Vol 95 (6) pp 1357–1364, https://doi.org/10.3945/ajcn.111.031070.

[166] EK Tarleton and B Littenberg (2015). 'Magnesium Intake and Depression in Adults.' *The Journal of the American Board of Family Medicine*. Vol 28 (2) pp 249–256. doi:10.3122/jabfm.2015.02.140176

[167] B Li, J Lv, W Wang et al. (2017). 'Dietary Magnesium and Calcium Intake and Risk of Depression in the General Population: A meta-analysis.' *Australian & New Zealand Journal of Psychiatry*. Vol 51 (3) p 219. https://doi.org/10.1177/0004867416676895

[168] EK Tarleton, B Littenberg, CD MacLean et al. (2017). 'Role of Magnesium Supplementation in the Treatment of Depression: A randomized clinical trial.' *PloS one*. Vol 12 (6), e0180067. doi:10.1371/journal.pone.0180067

[169] EK Tarleton, AG Kennedy, GL Rose et al. (2019). 'The Association between Serum Magnesium Levels and Depression in an Adult Primary Care Population.' *Nutrients*. Vol 11 (7) p 1475. doi:10.3390/nu11071475; A Serefko, A Szopa, P Wlaz et al. (2013). 'Magnesium in Depression.' *Pharmacological Reports*. Vol 65 pp 547–554; GA Eby and KL Eby (2006). 'Rapid Recovery From Major Depression Using Magnesium Treatment'. *Medical Hypotheses*. Vol 67 pp 362–370.

[170] FH Nielsen (2014). 'Effects of Magnesium Depletion on Inflammation in Chronic Disease.' *Current Opinion in Clinical Nutrition and Metabolic Care*. Vol 17 pp 525–530.

[171] G Grases, JA Perez-Castello, P Sanchis et al. (2006). 'Anxiety and Stress Among Science Students: Study of calcium and magnesium alterations.' *Magnesium Research*. Vol 19 pp 102–106; G Wanli, N Hussain, L Zongsuo et al. (2016). 'Magnesium Deficiency in Plants: An urgent problem.' *The Crop Journal*. Vol 4 (2) pp 83–91.

[172] J Gladd (2016). Alternative and Complementary Therapies. Vol 22 (4) http://doi. org/10.1089/act.2016.29068.jgl Accessed 2019.07.04

[173] J Wang, Y Liu, L Zhou et al (2009). 'Magnesium L-threonate Prevents and Restores Memory Deficits Associated with Neuropathic Pain by Inhibition of TNF-α.' *Pain Physician*. Vol 16 (5) pp 563–575.

[174] G Liu, JG Weinger, ZL Lu et al. (2016). 'Efficacy and Safety of MMFS-01, a Synapse Density Enhancer, for Treating Cognitive Impairment in Older Adults: A randomized, double-blind, placebo-controlled trial.' *Journal of Alzheimer's Disease: JAD*. Vol 49 (4) pp 971–990. doi:10.3233/JAD-150538

[175] W Swardfager, N Herrmann, RS McIntyre et al. (2013). 'Potential Roles of Zinc in the Pathophysiology and Treatment of Major Depressive Disorder'. *Neuroscience & Biobehavioral Reviews*. Vol 37 (5) pp 911–929; AS Prasad (1985). 'Clinical Manifestations of Zinc Deficiency.' *Annual Review of Nutrition*. Vol 5 (1) pp 341–363.

[176] P Enhui, Z Xiao-an, H Zhen et al. (2011). 'Vesicular Zinc Promotes Presynaptic and Inhibits Postsynaptic Long-Term Potentiation of Mossy Fiber-CA3 Synapse.' *Neuron*. Vol 71 (6) pp 1116–1126.

[177] O Dean, F Giorlando, M Berk (2011). 'N-acetylcysteine in Psychiatry: Current therapeutic evidence and potential mechanisms of action.' *Journal of Psychiatry & Neuroscience : JPN*. Vol 36 (2) pp 78–86. doi:10.1503/jpn.100057; JE Grant, BL Odlaug and SW Kim. (2009). 'N-acetylcysteine, a Glutamate Modulator, in the Treatment of Trichotillomania: A double-blind, placebo-controlled study.' *Archives of General Psychiatry*. Vol 66 pp 756–763; M Berk, DL Copolov, O Dean et al. (2008).

'N-acetylcysteine for Depressive Symptoms in Bipolar Disorder — A double-blind randomized placebo-controlled trial.' *Biological Psychiatry*. Vol 64 pp 468–475.

178 O Dean, F Giorlando and M Berk (2011). 'N-acetylcysteine in Psychiatry: Current therapeutic evidence and potential mechanisms of action.' *Journal of Psychiatry & Neuroscience: JPN*. Vol 36 (2) pp 78–86. doi:10.1503/jpn.100057

179 JS Deepmala, N Kumar, L Delhey et al. (2015). 'Clinical Trials of N-acetylcysteine in Psychiatry and Neurology: A systematic review.' *Neuroscience & Biobehavioral Reviews*. Vol 55 pp 294–321.

180 SL Ooi, R Green and SC Pak (2018) 'N-acetylcysteine for the Treatment of Psychiatric Disorders: A review of current evidence'. *BioMed Research International*. Vol 2018. doi: 10.1155/2018/2469486

181 F Javelle, A Lampit, W Bloch et al. (2019). 'Effects of 5-hydroxytryptophan on Distinct Types of Depression: A systematic review and meta-analysis'. *Nutrition Reviews*. Vol 78 (1) pp 77–88. https://doi.org/10.1093/nutrit/nuz039; KA Shaw, J Turner and C Del Mar. (2002). 'Tryptophan and 5-Hydroxytryptophan for Depression.' *Cochrane Database of Systematic Reviews*. Issue 1. Art. No.: CD003198. doi: 10.1002/14651858.CD003198.

182 J Jacobsen, AD Krystal, K Krishnan et al. (2016). 'Adjunctive 5-Hydroxytryptophan Slow-Release for Treatment-Resistant Depression: Clinical and preclinical rationale.' *Trends in Pharmacological Sciences*. Vol 37 (11) pp 933–944. doi:10.1016/j.tips.2016.09.001

183 A Sharma, P Gerbarg, T Bottiglieri et al. (2017) 'Work Group of the American Psychiatric Association Council on Research. S-Adenosylmethionine (SAMe) for Neuropsychiatric Disorders: A clinician-oriented review of research.' *The Journal of Clinical Psychiatry*. Vol 78 (6) pp 656–667. doi:10.4088/JCP.16r11113

184 WI Najm, S Reinsch, F Hoehler et al. (2004). 'S-adenosyl methionine (SAMe) Versus Celecoxib for the Treatment of Osteoarthritis Symptoms: A double-blind cross-over trial. [ISRCTN36233495].' *BMC Musculoskeletal Disorders*. Vol 5 p 6. doi:10.1186/1471-2474-5-6

185 D De Berardis, L Orsolini, N Serroni et al. (2016). 'A Comprehensive Review on the Efficacy of S-Adenosyl-L-methionine in Major Depressive Disorder. CNS & Neurological Disorders.' *Drug Targets*. Vol 15 p 35. https://doi.org/10.2174/18715 27314666150821103825

186 A Yoto, S Murao M Motoki, et al. (2012). 'Oral Intake of γ-aminobutyric Acid Affects Mood and Activities of Central Nervous System During Stressed Condition Induced by Mental Tasks.' *Amino Acids.* (2012) Vol 43 p 1331. https://doi.org/10.1007/s00726-011-1206-6

187 H Nakamura, T Takishima, T Kometani et al. (2009). 'Psychological Stress-reducing Effect of Chocolate Enriched with γ-aminobutyric Acid (GABA) in Humans: Assessment of stress using heart rate variability and salivary chromogranin.' *International Journal of Food Sciences and Nutrition.* Vol 60 (5) pp 106–113. DOI: 10.1080/09637480802558508

188 JI Byun, YY Shin, SE Chung et al. (2018). 'Safety and Efficacy of Gamma-Aminobutyric Acid from Fermented Rice Germ in Patients with Insomnia Symptoms: A randomized, double-blind trial.' *Journal of Clinical Neurology* (Seoul, Korea). Vol 14 (3) pp 291–295. doi:10.3988/jcn.2018.14.3.291

189 V Juturu, K Sahin, F Akdemir et al. (2016). 'M-A-T (Mucuna, Ashwagandha and Tribulus) Enhances Testosterone and Reduces Oxidative Stress: In vivo model.' *The FASEB Journal.* Vol 30 (1) supplement pp 404–404.

190 K Chandrasekhar, J Kapoor and S Anishetty (2012). 'A Prospective, Randomized Double-blind, Placebo controlled Study of Safety and Efficacy of a High-concentration Full Spectrum Extract of Ashwagandha Root in Reducing Stress and Anxiety in Adults.' *Indian Journal of Psychological Medicine.* Vol 34 pp 255–262.

191 B Auddy, J Hazra, A Mitra et al. (2008). 'A Standardized *Withania somnifera* Extract Significantly Reduces Stress-related Parameters in Chronically Stressed Humans: A double-blind, randomized, placebo-controlled study.' *Journal of the American Neutraceutical Association.* Vol 11 pp 50–56.

192 C Andrade, A Aswath, SK Chaturvedi et al. (2000). 'A Double-blind, Placebo-controlled Evaluation of the Anxiolytic Efficacy of an Ethanolic Extract of *Withania somnifera.*' *Indian Journal of Psychiatry.* Vol 42 (3) pp 295–301.

193 S Khyati and T B Anup (2013). 'A Randomized Double Blind Placebo Controlled Study of Ashwagandha on Generalized Anxiety Disorder.' *International Ayurvedic Medical Journal.* Vol 1 pp 1–7.

194 M Candelario, E Cuellar, J Mauricio Reyes-Ruiz et al. (2015). 'Direct Evidence for GABAergic Activity of *Withania somnifera* on Mammalian Ionotropic GABAA and GABAρ Receptors.' *Journal of Ethnopharmacology.* Vol 171 pp 264–272.

[195] K Cooley, O Szczurko, D Perri Mills et al. (2009). 'Naturopathic Care for Anxiety: A randomized controlled trial ISRCTN78958974.' *PloS One*. Vol 4 (8), e6628. doi:10.1371/journal.pone.0006628

[196] RH Singh, K Narsimhamurthy and G Singh (2008) 'Neuronutrient Impact of Ayurvedic Rasayana Therapy in Brain Aging.' *Biogerontology*. Vol 9 pp 369–374.

[197] V Viji and A Helen (2008). Inhibition of Lipoxygenases and Cyclooxygenase-2 enzymes by Extracts Isolated from *Bacopa monniera (L.) Wettst.' Journal of Ethnopharmacology*. Vol 118 (2) pp 305–311; P Jain, NK Khanna, N Trehan et al. (1994). 'Anti-inflammatory Effects of an Ayurvedic Preparation, Brahmi Rasayan, in Rodents.' *Indian Journal of Experimental Biology*. Vol 32 pp 633–636.

[198] D Kennedy, G Wake, S Savelev et al. (2003). 'Modulation of Mood and Cognitive Performance Following Acute Administration of Single Doses of *Melissa officinalis* (Lemon Balm) with Human CNS Nicotinic and Muscarinic Receptor-binding Properties.' *Neuropsychopharmacology*. Vol 28 pp 1871–1881. doi: 10.1038/sj.npp.1300230; DO Kennedy, W Little and AB Scholey (2004). 'Attenuation of Laboratory-induced Stress in Humans after Acute Administration of *Melissa officinalis* (Lemon Balm)'. *Psychosomatic Medicine*. Vol 66 pp 607–613. doi: 10.1097/01.psy.0000132877.72833.71.

[199] A Scholey, A Gibbs, C Neale et al. (2014). 'Anti-stress Effects of Lemon Balm-containing Foods. *Nutrients*. Vol 6 (11) pp 4805–4821. doi:10.3390/nu6114805

[200] O Turel, Q He, G Xue et al. (2014). 'Examination of Neural Systems Sub-Serving Facebook "Addiction."' *Psychological Reports*. Vol 115 (3) pp 675–695.

[201] BA Primack, A Shensa, JE Sidani et al. (2017). 'Social Media Use and Perceived Social Isolation Among Young Adults in the US.' *American Journal of Preventive Medicine*. Vol 53 (1) pp 1–8. doi:10.1016/j.amepre.2017.01.010

[202] https://newsroom.fb.com/news/2017/12/hard-questions-is-spending-time-on-social-media-bad-for-us/. Accessed 2019.07.21

[203] CK Ra, J Cho, MD Stone et al. (2018). 'Association of Digital Media Use With Subsequent Symptoms of Attention-Deficit/Hyperactivity Disorder Among Adolescents.' *Journal of the American Medical Association*. Vol 320 (3) pp 255–263. doi:10.1001/jama.2018.8931

[204] RJ van den Eijnden, GJ Meerkerk, AA Vermulst et al. (2008). 'Online Communication, Compulsive Internet Use, and Psychosocial Well-being Among

Adolescents: A longitudinal study.' *Developmental Psychology*. Vol 44 (3) pp 655–665.

205 D Greenfield (2012). 'The Addictive Properties of Internet Usage.' *Internet Addiction: A handbook and guide to evaluation and treatment* pp 135-153. 10.1002/9781118013991

206 American Psychological Association (2017). 'Stress in America: Coping with change.' *Stress in America™ Survey*. https://www.apa.org/news/press/releases/stress/2017/technology-social-media.pdf. Accessed 2019.8.12

207 B Primack, A Shensa, J Sidani et al. (2017). 'Social Media Use and Perceived Social Isolation Among Young Adults in the US.' *American Journal of Preventive Medicine*. Vol 53 (1) pp 1–8.

208 BA Primack, A Shensa, CG Escobar-Viera et al. (2017). 'Use of Multiple Social Media Platforms and Symptoms of Depression and Anxiety: A nationally-representative study among US young adults.' *Computers in Human Behavior*. Vol 69 pp 1–9.

209 A Vannucci, KM Flannery and CM Ohannessian (2017). 'Social Media Use and Anxiety in Emerging Adults.' *Journal of Affective Disorders*. Vol 207 pp 163–166.

210 JM Twenge, TE Joiner, ML Rogers et al. (2018). 'Increases in Depressive Symptoms, Suicide-Related Outcomes, and Suicide Rates Among US Adolescents After 2010 and Links to Increased New Media Screen Time.' *Clinical Psychological Science*. Vol 6 (1) pp 3–17.

211 HC Woods and H Scott (2016). '#Sleepyteens: Social media use in adolescence is associated with poor sleep quality, anxiety, depression and low self-esteem.' *Journal of Adolescence*. Vol 51 pp 41–49.

212 World of Chemicals (2019). 'Chemistry of Social Media Addiction.' *Kimberlite Softwares Pvt. Ltd, India*. https://www.worldofchemicals.com/512/chemistry-articles/chemistry-of-social-media-addiction.html. Accessed 2019.08.03

213 H Appel, AL Gerlach and J Crusius (2016). 'The Interplay Between Facebook Use, Social Comparison, Envy, and Depression.' *Current Opinion in Psychology*. Vol 9 pp 44–49.

214 M Lim (2018). 'Australian Psychological Society Australian Loneliness Report.' Analysis and Policy Observatory website: https://apo.org.au/node/202286. Accessed 2019.08.16

215 All things to do with Charlie Brown and the Peanuts comic strips are copyright Charles Schulz. https://thecharliebrown.tumblr.com/post/1632466498/charlie-brown-can-you-cure-loneliness-lucy-for/amp. Accessed 2019.09.25

216 LC Hawkley and JT Cacioppo (2010). 'Loneliness Matters: A theoretical and empirical review of consequences and mechanisms.' *Annals of Behavioral Medicine: A Publication of the Society of Behavioral Medicine.* Vol 40 (2) pp 218–227. doi:10.1007/s12160-010-9210-8

217 DM Tice and E Bratslavsky (2000). 'Giving in to Feel Good: The place of emotion regulation in the context of general self-control.' *Psychological Inquiry.* Vol 11 pp 149–159.

218 TD Geracioti (2006). 'Identifying Hypothyroidism's Psychiatric Presentations.' *Current Psychiatry.* Vol 5 (11) pp 98.

219 A Al-Heeti (2018). 'Voice Calls on Mobile Networks See First-ever Decline in UK.' https://www.cnet.com/news/thought-phone-calls-were-outdated-theyre-only-declining-now/. Accessed 2019.08.17

220 Wainwright M (2005). 'Emails "Pose Threat to IQ". Technology.' *The Guardian* https://www.theguardian.com/technology/2005/apr/22/money.workandcareers. Accessed 2019.08.03

221 KK Loh and R Kanai(2014). 'Higher Media Multi-Tasking Activity is Associated with Smaller Gray-Matter Density in the Anterior Cingulate Cortex'. *PLoS One.* Vol 9 (9) e106698. https://doi.org/10.1371/journal.pone.0106698

222 M Jackson (2014). 'The Stress of Life: A modern complaint?' *Lancet.* Vol 383 pp 300–301.

223 DR Samson, AN Crittenden, IA Mabulla et al. (2017). 'Hadza Sleep Biology: Evidence for flexible sleep-wake patterns in hunter-gatherers.' *American Journal of Physical Anthropology.* Vol 162 (3) pp 573–582.

224 R Ekirch (2005). *At Day's Close: Night in times past.* WW Norton & Company.

225 RE Roberts and HT Duong (2014). 'The Prospective Association Between Sleep Deprivation and Depression Among Adolescents.' *Sleep.* Vol 37 (2) pp 239–244. doi:10.5665/sleep.3388

226 RJ Havis (2018). 'The Surprising New Connection Between Sleep and Mental Health.' *Talk Space*. https://www.talkspace.com/blog/the-surprising-new-connection-between-sleep-and-mental-health/. Accessed 2019.08.01

227 L Xie, H Kang, Q Xu et al. (2013). 'Sleep Drives Metabolite Clearance from the Adult Brain.' *Science*. Vol 342 pp 373–377.

228 LM Lyall, CA Wyse, N Graham et al. (2018). 'Association of Disrupted Circadian Rhythmicity with Mood Disorders, Subjective Wellbeing, and Cognitive Function: A cross-sectional study of 91 105 participants from the UK Biobank.' *Lancet Psychiatry*. Vol 5 (6) pp 507–514. 10.1016/S2215-0366(18)30139-1

229 F Rutters, SG Lemmens, TC Adam et al. (2014). 'Is Social Jetlag Associated with an Adverse Endocrine, Behavioral, and Cardiovascular Risk Profile?' *Journal of Biological Rhythms*. Vol 29 (5) pp 377–383; RG Foster, SN Peirson, K Wulff et al. (2013). 'Sleep and Circadian Rhythm Disruption in Social Jetlag and Mental Illness.' In MU Gillette (ed). *Progress in Molecular Biology and Translational Science*. Academic Press. Vol 119 pp 325–346.

230 L Tähkämö, T Partonen and A K Pesonen (2019). 'Systematic Review of Light Exposure Impact on Human Circadian Rhythm.' *Chronobiology International*. Vol 36 (2) pp 151–170. doi: 10.1080/07420528.2018.1527773

231 SA Rahman, CM Shapiro, F Wang et al.(2013). 'Effects of Filtering Visual Short Wavelengths During Nocturnal Shiftwork on Sleep and Performance.' *Chronobiology International*. Vol 30 (8) pp 951–962. doi:10.3109/07420528.2013.7898 94

232 DF Kripke, RD Langer, JA Elliott et al. (2011). 'Mortality Related to Actigraphic Long and Short Sleep.' *Sleep Medicine*. Vol 12 (1) pp 28–33. doi:10.1016/j. sleep.2010.04.016

233 K Mikkelsen, L Stojanovska, M Polenakovic et al. (2017). 'Exercise and Mental Health.' *Maturitas*. Vol 106 pp 48–56.

234 F Dimeo, M Bauer, I Varahram et al. (2001). 'Benefits from Aerobic Exercise in Patients with Major Depression: A pilot study.' *British Journal of Sports Medicine*. Vol 35 (2) pp 114–117; AL Dunn, MH Trivedi and HA O'Neal (2001). 'Physical Activity Dose-response Effects on Outcomes of Depression and Anxiety.' *Medicine in Science and Sports and Exercise*. Vol 33 (6) pp 587–97.

[235] SB Harvey, S Øverland, SL Hatch et al. (2018). 'Exercise and the Prevention of Depression: Results of the HUNT Cohort Study.' *American Journal of Psychiatry*. Vol 17 pp 28–36.

[236] M Peluso and L Andrade (2005). 'Physical Activity and Mental Health: The association between exercise and mood.' *Clinics*. Vol 60 (1) pp 61–70. https://dx.doi.org/10.1590/S1807-59322005000100012

[237] J Firth, B Stubbs, D Vancampfort et al. (2018). 'Effect of Aerobic Exercise on Hippocampal Volume in Humans: A systematic review and meta-analysis.' *NeuroImage*. Vol 166 pp 230–238.

[238] S Dimitrov, E Hulteng and S Hong (2017). 'Inflammation and Exercise: Inhibition of monocytic intracellular TNF production by acute exercise via β2-adrenergic activation.' *Brain, Behavior, and Immunity*. Vol 61 pp 60–68.

[239] Mayo Clinic Staff (2017). 'Depression and Anxiety: Exercise eases symptoms.' *Mayo Clinic* https://www.mayoclinic.org/diseases-conditions/depression/in-depth/depression-and-exercise/art-20046495. Accessed 2019.07.10

[240] BT Heijmans, EW Tobi, AD Stein et al. (2008). 'Persistent Epigenetic Differences Associated with Prenatal Exposure to Famine in Humans.' *Proceedings of the National Academy of Sciences of the United States of America*. Vol 105 (44) pp 17046–17049; LO Bygren, P Tinghög, J Carstensen et al. (2014). 'Change in Paternal Grandmothers' Early Food Supply Influenced Cardiovascular Mortality of the Female Grandchildren.' *BMC Genetics*. Vol 15 p 12. doi:10.1186/1471-2156-15-12

[241] D Chopra, RE Tanzi (2015). *Super Genes: Unlock the astonishing power of your DNA for optimum health and wellbeing*. Harmony Books. p 31.

[242] J Bohacek and IM Mansuy (2015). 'Molecular Insights into Transgenerational Non-genetic Inheritance of Acquired Behaviours.' *Nature Reviews Genetics*. Vol 16 pp 641–652.

[243] R Zanca, S Braren, B Maloney et al (2015). 'Environmental Enrichment Increases Hippocampal Glucocorticoid Receptors and Decreases GluA2 and Protein Kinase M zeta (PKMz) Trafficking During Chronic Stress: A protective mechanism?' *Frontiers in Behavioral Neuroscience*. Vol 9 p 303.

[244] H Palma-Gudiel, A Córdova-Palomera, JC Leza et al. (2015). 'Glucocorticoid Receptor Gene (NR3C1) Methylation Processes as Mediators of Early Adversity in

Stress-related Disorders Causality: A critical review.' *Neuroscience & Biobehavioral Reviews*. Vol 55 pp 520–535.

245 JK McCreary and GAS Metz (2016). 'Environmental Enrichment as an Intervention for Adverse Health Outcomes of Prenatal Stress.' *Environmental Epigenetics*. Vol 2 (3).

246 A Lutz, HA Slagter, JD Dunne et al. (2008). 'Attention Regulation and Monitoring in Meditation.' *Trends in Cognitive Sciences*. Vol 12 (4) pp 163–169. doi:10.1016/j. tics.2008.01.005

247 M Metzler, G Metz and D Saucier (2013). 'Enriched Childhood Experiences Moderate Age-related Motor and Cognitive Decline.' *Frontiers in Behavioral Neuroscience*. Vol 7 p 1.

248 E Anderson and G Shivakumar (2013). 'Effects of Exercise and Physical Activity on Anxiety.' *Frontiers in Psychiatry*. Vol 4 p 27. doi:10.3389/fpsyt.2013.00027

249 F Williams (2016). 'Call to the Wild: This is your brain on nature.' *National Geographic*. https://www.nationalgeographic.com/magazine/2016/01/call-to-wild/. Accessed 2019.06.02.

250 C Sarkar, C Webster and J Gallacher (2018). 'Residential Greenness and Prevalence of Major Depressive Disorders: A cross-sectional, observational, associational study of 94 879 adult UK Biobank participants.' *The Lancet Planetary Health*. Vol 2 (4) pp 162–173.

251 BJ Park, Y Tsunetsugu, T Kasetani et al. (2010). 'The Physiological effects of Shinrin-yoku (Taking in the Forest Atmosphere or Forest Bathing): Evidence from field experiments in 24 forests across Japan.' *Environmental Health and Preventive Medicine*. Vol 15 (1) pp 18–26. doi:10.1007/s12199-009-0086-9

252 I Buric, M Farias, J Jong et al. (2017). 'What is the Molecular Signature of Mind–Body Interventions? A systematic review of gene expression changes induced by meditation and related practices.' *Frontiers in Immunology*. Vol 8 p 670.

253 P Kaliman, MJ Alvarez-López, M Cosín-Tomás Rosenkranz et al. (2014). 'Rapid Changes in Histone Deacetylases and Inflammatory Gene Expression in Expert Meditators.' *Psychoneuroendocrinology*. Vol 4 pp 96–107. doi:10.1016/j. psyneuen.2013.11.004

254 M Ravnik-Glavač, S Hrašovec, JB Jurij Dreu et al. (2012). 'Genome-wide Expression Changes in a Higher State of Consciousness.' *Consciousness and*

Cognition. Vol 21 (3) pp 1322–1344, ISSN 1053-8100. https://doi.org/10.1016/j. concog.2012.06.003

255 W Youyou, D Stillwell, HA Schwartz et al. (2017). 'Birds of a Feather Do Flock Together: Behavior-based personality-assessment method reveals personality similarity among couples and friends.' *Psychological Science.* Vol 28 (3) pp 276–284.

256 https://www.inc.com/peter-economy/oprah-winfrey-19-inspiring-power-quotes-for-success.html. Accessed 2019.08.12

257 ES Shuckburgh (trans) *Letters of Marcus Tullius Cicero.* Macmillan and Co.

PART 3: TOOLS TO ENRICH

258 C Boeree (2006). 'Viktor Frankl 1905–1997. Personality theories.' Shippensburg University. https://webspace.ship.edu/cgboer/frankl.html. Accessed 2019.10.20.

259 Viktor E Frankl (1959). *Man's Search for Meaning.* Beacon Press, p 66.

260 Robert L Wilson was elected to the Illinois House of Representatives and was a member of the 'Long Nine' of Whig assemblymen of Sangamon County. Abraham Lincoln was also a member of the party and the pair became friends. http://www. mrlincolnandfriends.org/the-politicians/robert-wilson/

261 S Blumenthal (2016). *A Self Made Man: The political life of Abraham Lincoln.* Vol 1, 1809–1849. Simon and Schuster, New York.

262 Abraham Lincoln (1809–1865). *Collected Works of Abraham Lincoln.* Volume 5. [online] 2019. https://quod.lib.umich.edu/l/lincoln/lincoln5/1:643?rgn=div1;view=fulltext

263 AS Waterman, SJ Schwartz, BL Zamboanga et al. (2010). The Questionnaire for Eudaimonic Well-Being: Psychometric properties, demographic comparisons, and evidence of validity. *The Journal of Positive Psychology.* Vol 5 (1) pp 41–61.

264 C Papageorgiou and A Wells (2003). 'An Empirical Test of a Clinical Metacognitive Model of Rumination and Depression.' *Cognitive Therapy and Research.* Vol 27 p 261.

265 Lemony Snicket (1999). *A Series of Unfortunate Events. The bad beginning.* Harper Collins Publishers p 1.

266 R Razzaque (2014). *Breaking Down is Waking Up: The connection between psychological distress and spiritual awakening.* Watkins Publishing.

267 S Young (2004). *Break Through Pain: A step-by-step mindfulness meditation program for transforming chronic and acute pain.* Sounds True.

268 MD Lieberman, NI Eisenberger, MJ Crockett et al. (2007). 'Putting Feelings into Words: Affect labeling disrupts amygdala activity in response to affective stimuli.' *Psychological Science.* Vol 18 pp 421–428.

269 These emotions are viewed as negative and are undesired, as they make us extraordinarily uncomfortable. However, labelling emotions as negative creates resistance to that emotion. It is fine to feel anger, sadness, shame or vulnerability and these emotions should be felt without judgement.

270 JI Rosenberg (2019). *90 Seconds to a Life you Love.* Hachette.

271 RS Sneed and S Cohen (2013). 'A Prospective Study of Volunteerism and Hypertension Risk in Older Adults.' *Psychology and Aging.* Vol 28 (2) pp 578–586. doi:10.1037/a0032718

272 CE Jenkinson, AP Dickens, K Jones et al. (2013). 'Is Volunteering a Public Health Intervention? A systematic review and meta-analysis of the health and survival of volunteers.' *BioMed Central Public Health.* Vol 13 p 773. doi:10.1186/1471-2458-13-773

273 EW Dunn, LB Aknin and MI Norton (2008). 'Spending Money on Others Promotes Happiness.' *Science.* Vol 319 pp 1687–1688; SK Nelson, K Layous, SW Cole et al. (2016). 'Do Unto Others or Treat Yourself? The effects of prosocial and self-focused behavior on psychological flourishing.' *Emotion.* Vol 16 (6) pp 850–861. doi:10.1037/emo0000178. PMID: 27100366.

274 J Chancellor, S Margolis, BK Jacobs et al. (2018). 'Everyday Prosociality in the Workplace: The reinforcing benefits of giving, getting, and glimpsing.' *Emotion.* Vol 18 pp 507–517. 10.1037/emo0000321

275 D Kurt (2019). 'Are You in the Top One Percent of the World?' *Investopedia.* https://www.investopedia.com/articles/personal-finance/050615/are-you-top-one-percent-world.asp. Accessed 2019.09.20.

276 CN Armenta, MM Fritz, S Lyubomirsk (2017). 'Functions of Positive Emotions: Gratitude as a motivator of self-improvement and positive change. *Emotion Review.* Vol 9 (3) pp 183–190. https://doi.org/10.1177/1754073916669596

[277] ME McCullough, RA Emmons, JA Tsang (2002). 'The Grateful Disposition: A conceptual and empirical topography.' *Journal of Personality and Social Psychology.* Vol 82 (1) pp 112–127. https://doi.org/10.1037//0022-3514.82.1.112; JJ Froh, TB Kashdan, KM Ozimkowski et al. (2009). 'Who Benefits the Most From a Gratitude Intervention in Children and Adolescents? Examining positive affect as a moderator.' *The Journal of Positive Psychology.* Vol 4 (5) pp 408–422; PL Hill and M Allemand (2011). 'Gratitude, Forgivingness, and Well-being in Adulthood: Tests of moderation and incremental prediction.' *The Journal of Positive Psychology.* Vol 6 (5) pp 397–407. https://doi.org/10.1080/17439760.2011 .602099

[278] ME McCullough and RA Emmons (2003). 'Counting Blessings Versus Burdens.' *Journal of Personality and Social Psychology.* Vol 84 (2) pp 377–89.

[279] S Allen (2018). *The Science of Gratitude.* Greater Good Science Center UC Berkley. https://ggsc.berkeley.edu/images/uploads/GGSC-JTF_White_Paper-Gratitude-FINAL.pdf. Accessed 2019.06.21

[280] M Koo, SB Algoe,TD Wilson et al. (2008). 'It's a Wonderful Life: Mentally subtracting positive events improves people's affective states, contrary to their affective forecasts.' *Journal of Personality and Social Psychology.* Vol 95 (5) pp 1217–1224. https://doi.org/10.1037/a0013316

Index